Clinical Applications of Microcomputers
in Communication Disorders

SPEECH, LANGUAGE, AND HEARING

A Series of Monographs and Texts

NORMAN J. LASS

Department of Speech Pathology and Audiology
West Virginia University
Morgantown, West Virginia

Clinical Applications of Microcomputers in Communication Disorders

JAMES L. FITCH

Department of Speech Pathology and Audiology
College of Allied Health Professions
University of South Alabama
Mobile, Alabama

1986

ACADEMIC PRESS, INC.
Harcourt Brace Jovanovich, Publishers
Orlando   San Diego   New York   Austin
Boston   London   Sydney   Tokyo   Toronto

318162

ACADEMIC PRESS, INC.
Orlando, Florida 32887

United Kingdom Edition published by
ACADEMIC PRESS INC. (LONDON) LTD.
24–28 Oval Road, London NW1 7DX

Library of Congress Cataloging in Publication Data

Fitch, James L.
   Clinical applications of microcomputers in communication disorders.

   (Speech, language & hearing)
   Bibliography: p.
   Includes index.
   1. Communicative disorders—Data processing.
2. Microcomputers. I. Title. II. Series.
[DNLM: 1. Communicative Disorders—therapy. 2. Computer
Assisted Instruction. 3. Computers. WL 340 F545c]
RC429.F55 1986   616.85'5   86-3467
ISBN 0–12–257755–8 (hardcover) (alk. paper)
ISBN 0–12–257756–6 (paperback) (alk. paper)

PRINTED IN THE UNITED STATES OF AMERICA

86 87 88 89   9 8 7 6 5 4 3 2 1

Contents

Contents vii

12 Developing Software

13 The Future

Preface

The purpose of this book is to provide the reader with a comprehensive reference for the utilization of the microcomputer in the field of communication disorders. The book is appropriate as a text for courses on clinical management, as a reference book for the practicing professional, and as an information source for persons who have an interest in, or a need to stay current with, developments in the clinical management of communication disorders. The appendixes include a list of publishers of software for communication disorders, a suggested list of periodicals, and several utility programs which users can key into their own computers.

The book is designed to be readable by individuals with different levels of expertise in computer use. The novice who wants a comprehensive overview will want to read the complete book. However, individuals with special interests will find it more efficient to read selected chapters. The book is written in a manner that allows reading individual chapters without losing context.

Chapter 1 is a historical perspective of the computer in society and its role in the field of communication disorders. Chapter 2 deals with information needed to understand how computer hardware works. It is written in nontechnical terms; however, a glossary is available at the end of the book which will permit the reader to become familiar with common computer terminology. Chapter 3 discusses computer software. Computer languages are described with examples written in BASIC for the reader to consider. At the completion of Chapter 3 is an important section on guidelines for evaluating software. Chapter 4 presents the challenge that society faces in learning to live with technology.

Chapters 5 and 6 present an introduction to word processing and data management. Again, it is written in nontechnical terms and includes discussions of practical applications for professionals in the field. Specific examples of how to use word and data processing to write reports, maintain records, and enhance accountability of clinical operations are provided. These can serve as a basis for professionals to choose and develop computer programs and systems which are most appropriate in their own settings.

Chapters 7, 8, and 9 present a discussion of current specific applications of the computer to the field of speech–language pathology. Chapters 10 and 11 accomplish the same for specific applications in audiology. Programs that are commercially available and programs that are in the public domain are reviewed.

Chapter 12 is included for the individual who is interested in developing software for the field. There are a growing number of professionals in the field of communication disorders who are aware of the need for software development and who have the requisite computer skills. This chapter will help those understand what is needed to succeed as a professional software developer.

Chapter 13 paints a picture of the clinic of the future and the role that will be played by the computer. It is for the clinician who wants to look ahead to the needs of the future and learn how to prepare for them.

This book is the result of 15 years of experience with computers. During this time the author has found computers to be useful, fascinating, and fun. His goal in writing this book will have been met if it in some measure helps the reader to have a similar experience.

1
Perspective

We are in the midst of a technological revolution which is changing the landscape of our clinical fields. Clinical service delivery systems are now being developed which require quite different assumptions regarding the clinical process and how we can train students to engage in that process.

We are in an era where digital logic circuits are reshaping the potentials for clinical diagnosis and clinical management processes in very dramatic ways. Juxtapose that idea with the fact that most clinical fields change slowly. If the technology continues to advance at breakneck speed, then deliverers of clinical services either must develop sufficient knowledge about these devices so they can be utilized toward goals which are clinically sound, or the practitioners will become slaves to someone else's technology and lose control over the direction of the clinical process. (Minifie, 1981, p. 2)

The above is an excerpt from the keynote address to the National Council of Graduate Programs in Speech and Language Pathology and Audiology in 1981. It was the first major address to verbalize concern for the utilization of technology in clinical services in our field. Dr. Minifie's interest and influence in this area were evident throughout his tenure as President of the American Speech–Language–Hearing Association (ASHA). The 1983 ASHA Convention (over which Dr. Minifie presided) in Cincinnati had over 40 activities (short courses, technical sessions, exhibits, etc.) on the clinical application of computers. This was more than all of the previous ASHA Convention programs combined.

Support for dissemination of information on computer technology at a national level was also provided in 1983 when the American Speech–Language–Hearing Foundation (ASHF) adopted as a major project a conference on microcomputers. This conference, the Personal Computer as a Clinical Tool, was held in February 1984. It was one of the most important professional development opportunities to be afforded persons in the field of communication disorders concerning the clinical application of microcomputers. And it established computer applications as an integral component of curricula in the field of communication disorders. A second conference was sponsored by ASHF in 1985. The target audience for this conference was individuals with intermediate and advanced computer skills, reflecting the increasing level of training in the field.

COMPUTERS IN OTHER FIELDS

Computers have been an integral part of society almost from their inception. The first commercial computer, UNIVAC I, placed into operation in 1951, cost $12,000,000 to develop, filled a room, and required temperature and humidity control (Holoien, 1977). Today one can buy a personal computer for less than $1000 that has more memory, computes faster, and can sit on top of an ordinary desk. If the automotive industry had undergone comparable price and efficiency breakthroughs, a Rolls-Royce today would cost less than $3.00 and go 180,000 miles on a gallon of gas.

Business

Business was quick to apply the computer, obviously because the strength of the computer was most evident in its ability to manipulate numbers quickly. To draw the comparison between arithmetic computation of man and computer, consider the problem below.

$$
\begin{array}{r}
1625 \\
3329 \\
4184 \\
4996 \\
9215 \\
8317 \\
7632 \\
7518 \\
6040 \\
\underline{5051}
\end{array}
$$

To add as many of these problems as a computer can do in 1 second, a man would have to work 8 hours per day, 52 weeks per year for 133 years (Holoien, 1977).

Because of the speed with which the computer can manage numbers, the field of accounting embraced this technology with understandable enthusiasm. Computers are an integral part of the accounting field today. Almost all bills and bank statements you receive today are printed by a computer.

As fields change, people have to update skills to maintain job status. Universities today include a heavy dose of computing in accounting programs; in some cases it is difficult to determine whether the accounting major is an accounting major or a computer science major. Seminars on computer hardware and software applications are a part of the continuing education of accountants in the field.

Marketing is an area of business that has also been affected significantly by the computer. Since the marketing process is dependent upon consumers' current and future purchasing plans, consumer surveys are frequently conducted to determine purchasing patterns. The value of the computer is found in its ability to take the information from the survey and process it systematically. Survey data can be broken down statistically to provide the business with the information it needs to know about the consumer according to geographic location, socioeconomic status, sex, occupation, etc.

Surveys are also taken after the sale is made to determine customer satisfaction. The results of these surveys can be again processed by the computer and provide the seller with information needed to improve the product.

Surveys, plus records of buying habits of individuals, often form the basis for mailing lists. Promotion of a product by mail has become popular because it is an inexpensive, effective means of reaching the consumer directly. The words "You may have already won our sweepstakes, Mrs. _____" have become a part of our culture. The personalization that can be accomplished by using the computer allows the user to generate letters to "individuals" as fast as the printer can function.

Recently, management has incorporated the computer into the decision-making process. The computer can process information more quickly and accurately and decisions by management concerning the operation of a business are most effective when based on information that is current and accurate. The consolidation of the pertinent information about a business into a common file is analogous to having a "database" (Laver, 1980). Data-based management programs and electronic spreadsheets for computers are now among the most frequently purchased software. With recent improvements, not only do businesses have current information at hand, but they can manipulate it in a "what if?" game to project future needs. For example, a company can project what their needs for raw materials, labor, shipping, and other parts of their operation would be if they were to experience a 10% growth in sales. Through the use of a spreadsheet, all of the figures change nearly instantaneously when a single figure is changed.

Direct sales have also been affected by the computer. Often the "cash register" at the checkout counter is a computer terminal. It not only makes change, but also accepts information about the product which helps the store to keep track of inventory and know when to order merchandise that is moving well. Many supermarkets and department stores have scanning devices which can read the Universal Product Code from product labels. With the price and product identification coded into the computer, the checkout person merely passes the product label over the scanning device. The computer does the rest without the clerk having to punch a number. The result has been more accurate bills and faster service through the checkout lines (Logsdon, 1980).

Japan has been developing a system of computerized supermarket shopping through use of vending machines. Shoppers take a plastic shopping card when entering the store. Food is stored in vending machines which can be operated by inserting the card. Each insertion records the purchase in a central computer. At the checkout lane the clerk inserts the card in a terminal and a record of the purchases is printed. It is reported that this type of shopping reduces time in the checkout lane by a factor of seven (Logsdon, 1980).

Banking

Electronic Funds Transfer Systems (EFTS) are currently in development. The notion of a "cashless" society—the plastic card becoming the primary focal point of financial transactions—has existed for years (Logsdon, 1980). The concept of EFT is attractive in that the individual, and his bank, would know at any moment the current balance of his account. If a standard terminal was available to communicate with bank computers via telephone lines, transactions could be recorded from any place with telephone connections. It would eliminate the problem of outstanding checks and the inconvenience of delayed transactions.

Large-scale attempts at EFTS have been resisted, however, by both the bank and the customer. Banks have found they can actually lose money by adopting such a system. The speed of transactions using EFTS causes interest to be lost on the money that would normally remain under their control during the longer transfer delay period that exists with paper checks.

Resistance from the customer appears to come from the fear of loss of control. The traditional check writing schema appears to offer the customer, at the present time, better control over the process. For example, under the present system a customer can write a check that overdraws his account on the weekend, knowing he can put funds into the bank to cover it on Monday morning. EFTS would detect the overdraft immediately.

Many banks do have electronic funds transfer as a service to customers who wish to have it. In the present situation, people may pay bills by coding information to the computer via touch-tone telephone. The increase in postal costs will likely make the alternative of EFTS more attractive over time.

Politics

Although not as visible on a daily basis, the gains made by business in the use of the computer are paralleled by gains in the political arena. Politicians are subject to the wishes of constituents, which can range in number from thousands to millions. To maintain contact with the people they represent, many politicians maintain mailing lists on computers which permit them to prepare and distribute quickly and inexpensively surveys and information newsletters. For purposes of survival, politicians must also be able to reach the people who will vote at election time and determine their preferences. While widespread use of the media is most noticeable in this effort, direct mail campaigning is also an integral part of winning campaign efforts.

The computer has also made it possible for politicians to maintain additional mailing lists which identify recipients by age, occupation, geographic area, socioeconomic status and special interests. Through the computer, form letters can be generated which will address each characteristic of the individual to whom it was sent. As in all situations involving the computer, the work could have been done by hand. However, to type the 27,000,000 computer-generated letters that the Nixon campaign sent in 1972 (Holoien, 1977) would have required 1000 expert typists typing 8 hours per day, 5 days per week, for over a year.

Military

The military is perhaps even more dependent on the computer. Our primary source of defense and retaliation is missile warfare. While the amount of damage that can be inflicted by a missile carrying a nuclear warhead has never been in doubt, the accuracy of the missile to the target has been suspect. A few foreign particles on the surface of a missile traveling long distances can alter its course to the point that it is militarily meaningless. Through computerized feedback systems, missiles are now capable of almost absolute accuracy (Logsdon, 1980).

Virtually all phases of the military are dependent on computers for the national defense. Computers calculate trajectories for artillery and armor units, computer-enhanced reconnaissance photographs detect defense buildups, and computer simulation is used as supplementary training aids in many areas, notably flight training.

Medicine

Initially only the business operations of hospitals were computerized, with the result being quicker and easier check-in and check-out for patients and more efficient processing of insurance claims. Now, however, the computer has pervaded all aspects of the hospital operation. Nurses use computers to maintain patient reports in some centers. Pharmaceutical records on computers can save patient lives by quickly identifying drugs to which the patient has reactions. Blood and tissue testing can be done under computer control. Computer-enhanced tomography/radiology can provide more detailed visual results to locate site of lesion.

Computers can be interfaced with physiological sensors and programmed to signal the nurses' station when significant deviations in vital signs occur. Even brain surgery has found a use for the computer in determining the site of lesion (Holoien, 1977).

The computer can be used as a decision-making, or perhaps more accurately, decision-checking tool for physicians. The computer can be programmed to analyze a set of symptoms and suggest possible maladies and/ or recommend further tests to administer. Because many people in the field of communication disorders work in medical settings, more applications pertinent to the field will be found and the need to be current will become increasingly important.

Industry

Industry gives us perhaps the most important lesson in adapting to technology. Few people would argue that machines have changed our world in positive ways. They produce materials to build homes, ventilation systems to maintain temperatures in those homes, devices to prepare foods, means of transportation of people and goods, and countless other conveniences. Books could not be produced for mass consumption until the printing press. Radio and television created a niche in society for all forms of expression. The automobile and the airplane provided the power for reducing distance and changed our world. Few people would want to return to the days before these products.

Since the first machine to replace man was developed, however, there has been a Luddite psychology (attacking technology because it replaces human workers) accompanying every major technological advance. Machines replacing people means some people will lose their jobs. That is the price that must be paid and society does not seem to have coped well with that reality. In the past 200 years the civilized world has moved from muscle power to machine power. There is no reason to believe that this trend will be reversed.

In recent years we have seen the computer become an integral part of the printing industry. Typesetting, an occupation with a 400-year history, came virtually to an end when computers were programmed to accomplish the task. Many younger newspaper journalists have never worked on typewriters. They have known only the word processor in the preparation of material, since through it articles can be prepared and entered directly into the computer.

The example which perhaps should be considered most seriously is the development of robotics in the automobile industry. In the early days, workers protested that robots would be developed to do jobs traditionally done by men. This was deemed unacceptable because it would put men out of work. Japan, and other countries, however, embraced the new technology and used it to their advantage. For several years cars built in the United States could not compete with foreign cars. The choices were to (1) buy a car built by robots that could put a white-hot rivet in place wih a .01-inch tolerance; or (2) buy a car built by a man whose job was protected by a union, regardless of performance. In a free society, the common good usually wins out over special interests. The public's response to the automobile industry resulted in hundreds of thousands of workers being laid off their jobs. The situation is different today. United States companies incorporated robots into the production line and men went back to work. Not as many men are now working as before, but if the industry had not made the change when it did, there might not be an automobile industry in the United States today.

Computer-assisted design (CAD) and computer-assisted manufacturing (CAM) have become important tools in industry. Through computer simulation, designs can be tested before they are constructed. The design is tested against known parameters, allowing the designer to see what is going to happen without having to construct an expensive prototype. Computer control of the manufacturing process increases efficiency and quality control. Industrial usage of the computer is necessary for survival.

COMPUTERS IN COMMUNICATION DISORDERS

It has been suggested that the initial response to any kind of technology is generally adverse (Laver, 1980). Quite simply, people who are not trained feel that the new technology may replace them. In addition, there is a certain mystery in how the new technology works, and this lack of knowledge of what it is all about is discomforting to many. Then there is the natural inertia, the resistance to change, that causes people to view new developments with skepticism.

It should be remembered that all of the problems noted above are transient. Once the technology is in place, the people trained, and the concepts accepted, those problems disappear.

Those who work with communication disorders should continue to extend themselves to know and understand developments in other fields. Many other professions in our society have already incorporated the computer into their daily routine to a greater extent than we have. By examining the uses to which they have put the computer, and by studying the mistakes they have made, we should be in a better position to understand and control the emergence of this technology in our field.

There are positive signs that the field of communication disorders is, in fact, making the necessary effort to become current. First, the increased number of presentations at Annual ASHA Conventions in recent years indicates that many developments in many areas are in progress. It is also an indication that practioners are now interested in incorporating the computer into clinical activities. The American Speech–Language–Hearing Foundation's 1984 Conference on the Personal Computer as a Tool suggested that leaders in the field were aware of the need for professional development in that area. And the number of training programs including computer coursework as a part of their curriculum is increasing. The following statement by Minifie (1981) was both prophetic and directive:

> Electronic computers and other digital devices simply must become an integral part of our graduate education programs. That can only occur if we and our faculties master computer usage and adapt computers to our needs. Just as is true in the case of high school seniors, a course in computer programming or computer operation will not provide university instructors with the requisite skills and understandings. University teachers must first learn to use computers in the same manner that their students should subsequently learn to use them. (p. 7)

Students completing many of the training programs today that require computer literacy may wonder what the computer "revolution" is about. Many of them have already come to know and use the computer as a friendly tool. As in the case of industry, it is not the new workers with new skills who feel out of place; rather it is the workers who were trained and on the job before the new technology arrived who find themselves uncomfortable.

Recognizing the Need

In 1980 this author was appointed Chairman of the American Speech–Language–Hearing Association's Committee on Educational Technology. The project of the first year of that appointment was a survey of emerging technology. It was found that over 80% of new technological developments in the field had to do with computers (Fitch, 1981). The next project of the Committee was to identify computer programs which were being developed. This lead to the publication of the first edition of the Software Registry (Fitch, 1982). When it became evident that computers were going to become an integral part of the clinical scene, there was an element of panic in inquiries to the Committee. The question that was heard most often in 1981 was "Will the computer replace me?" It was accompanied by a real fear that technology was about to erode the already tightening job market for specialists in communication disorders.

As of this writing, the response to technology has changed 180 degrees. Instead of the question "Will computers replace me?" the question now is "Will someone who knows how to use a computer replace me?" In many cases the answer is already "maybe." Some educational programs are now requiring employees to take coursework and develop competency in working with computers. Many professionals in schools, hospitals, and universities are finding that other professionals are using computers and that their own service is being questioned as to why they are not. This will become more acute as the younger population grows up with computers and accepts them as an integral part of their lives. Minifie (1981) expressed it in the following manner:

> Maybe you hope to keep computers at a distance by dealing with them only at work or trying to escape them altogether. There is no such escape. They are already invading our homes as pocket calculators or electronic games, may be lurking in the controls of our microwave ovens, and soon will evidence themselves in television sets that respond to our spoken commands. Our popular magazines now regularly carry large advertisements for the so-called "home" or "personal" computers that enable us, as well as others, to keep on file more information than we can comprehend. If you do not think that you regularly communicate with computers, examine your in and out mail for today. Chances are that more of it came from computers than people, and that a computer is the ultimate destination for most of your missives. (p. 3)

It would seem that the issue now is not whether, but how, to get involved in computers. Based on observation, personal experience and reports of many persons in the field making the transition, the following general principles are suggested.

Attitude

The first, and most important, consideration in coping with the computer is attitude. Luddite antagonism and technological panic are counterproductive. Perhaps the most productive attitude has its foundation in remembering always that the clinician is the critical element in treatment. The computer is a tool, a powerful one if used wisely, but still a tool and only useful under the guidance of a clinician.

A second consideration having to do with attitude is patience. It is probably true that most clinicians will need to know something about the computer. However, no one is going to expect them to learn everything at one time. Occasionally participants in workshops for beginners are frustrated because they did not learn all that they felt they needed to know at that time. It must be remembered that even the programs that are supposedly "user-friendly" take time to master. Secretaries who work daily with a word processing program find that after a year they are still learning new things that it can do. Computers and programs take time to learn. Clinicians should realize that learning the computer will be a process that will probably continue throughout their careers. New programs and new equipment capable of more sophisticated communications will continue to emerge, challenging us to find new uses.

The last point to consider regarding attitude is control. At this point many professionals feel that the computer is in control—that they are dependent on what it can do and what it can be programmed to do. The clinician should approach the task of learning a computer with the same attitude that is necessary for driving an automobile. The goal is not merely to operate the machine, but to be able to control it to make it do what you want it to do. A car may be able to move at a rate of speed in excess of 100 miles per hour, but few people would exercise that option. The computer may have incredible power and versatility, but it is meaningless if clinicians cannot make it do what they want it to do.

Professional Development Planning

The proper attitude will lead to a plan of professional development that will result in usable computer skills. It is important for clinicians to include plans for developing computer skills in their professional development program. Again, one should be cautioned not to try to learn it all at one time. The plan should evolve over a period of time and be less pressured.

In developing skill with the computer, the most important part of training is hands-on experience. Nothing can replace the experience of sitting at, and interacting with, a computer. Computers are devices which epitomize the adage that "you learn by your mistakes." Computers do not penalize for mistakes. Trial and error is an acceptable, even desirable, method of learning on the computer. When learning a new program, even experienced computer users sometimes try different things just to see what will happen.

A second strategy for learning computers is to obtain instruction from as many different settings as possible. Computer stores often have introduction seminars. Do not stop with one seminar; take all that are available. Universities, 2-year community colleges, and vocational schools often have good, practical courses. One precaution: when taking a formal computer course, check ahead to ensure that there is sufficient hands-on experience and that the ratio of students to computers is no greater than two to one. The same is true of workshops and conferences. Unless there is special purpose information which can be learned through traditional lecture, make sure that demonstration and training components are included.

Part of Professional Development

Last, learning a new skill takes some dedication and investment of time, energy, and money. One of the best investments, perhaps even the best, that a professional in any field can make today is in computers. The rewards for being able to use a computer increase as skill in using it increases. And the relationship is more logarithmic than linear.

BENEFITS OF COMPUTER POWER

Reduced Paperwork

The primary benefit of the computer is efficiency in handling paperwork. In a time in which accountability and documentation have become a way of life, the computer offers a means of welcome relief. For persons who are required to write diagnostic and progress reports and those who are required to file Individual Treatment Plans (ITPS) or Individual Educational Plan (IEPS) the computer can be an exceptionally helpful tool. For example, the most detailed report should require no more than 15 minutes from start to finish, including proofreading and printing the report on a printer. ITPs should require even less time, given the use of an efficient program.

More Time for Clinical Activities

The efficiency one gains in paperwork translates into more time for the clinical activities themselves. Using the computer to write reports does not save time in the clinical diagnostic process itself. Actually, knowing that the diagnostic report is going to take less time to write generally encourages the clinician to take more time in the diagnostic session itself.

Utilization of Support Personnel

The use of the computer in the direct delivery of services also increases the efficiency of the clinician. Because screening and treatment procedures can be under computer control, it is possible to utilize support personnel to administer the drill and practice type of exercises. Programs that present stimuli and store responses can also relieve the clinician of counting and recording responses. This allows the clinician to concentrate on the client and the behavior itself more fully.

Direct Patient–Computer Treatment

Clinical programs which interact directly with the client are also beneficial. These are usually supplemental drill and practice exercises. The practice can be done at home or in the clinic, but does not require the clinician to be present at all times. This obviously is a cost-efficient type of treatment. There also may be psychological advantages to the client interacting with the computer since it fosters independence and is nonjudgmental (Fitch & Cross, 1983). Thus, the computer may meet the needs of a particular client better than a clinician. This will be discussed in more detail in Chapter 9.

Professional Image

The image projected from the provision of computer-based services is a positive one. People expect computer applications in most fields and the field that does not utilize it suffers a credibility gap. If the field of communication disorders is to project a respected professional image, technology must be adopted.

Better Care for the People Served

The most important consideration in utilizing computers in clinical services is whether the computer offers hope that better care can be offered to the people served. If by incorporating computers into their practices, clinicians can make themselves more efficient and their services more cost effective, and they can provide supplemental services which work to the betterment of the people served, then it should be done. After all, providing the best services possible is a goal that should be sought by each clinician.

SUMMARY

There are landmark developments in the history of man which are of such significance that they cannot be ignored. The computer is one of those landmark developments. What the machine did for human muscle, the computer does for the mind. Fields such as industry and business, which must stay competitive globally, have embraced the electronic technology and through it have reached new heights.

As a profession, the field of communication disorders must realize the need for computer utilization and take measures to ensure the development of computer skills. There must be a commitment by the profession as a whole, and a commitment by individuals. The field is faced with a time of great challenge and even greater opportunity. How we respond to that challenge will have a significant impact upon our future.

References

Fitch, J. (1981). *Report of Committee on Educational Technology.* American Speech–Language–Hearing Association Committee on Educational Technology, Rockville, MD.

Fitch, J. (Ed.) (1982). *Software registry* (1st ed.). American Speech–Language–Hearing Association Committee on Educational Technology, Rockville, MD.

Fitch, J., & Cross, S. (1983). Telecomputer treatment of aphasia. *Journal of Speech and Hearing Disorders,* **48,** 335–336.

Holoien, M. (1977). *Computers and their societal impact.* New York: Wiley.

Laver, M. (1980). *Computers and social change.* Cambridge, MA: Cambridge University Press.

Logsdon, T. (1980). *Computers and social controversy.* Potomac, MD: Computer Science Press.

Minifie, F. (1981). Graduate education during a technological revolution. *National Council of Graduate Programs in Speech and Language Pathology and Audiology Proceedings,* Rockville, MD, pp. 1–9.

2

Hardware

Basic computer configurations include four components; input, processor, storage, and output (Fig. 1). The heart and soul of the system is the processor. It accepts information, integrates and manipulates it, and can perform logical operations on it. However, the processor alone is useless. Like the human brain, it can reach its full potential only if it has a meaningful flow of information to it. And it can impact on the world only to the degree to which it can communicate its findings to the outside world.

This chapter will discuss the components individually and in a manner that is intended to communicate to the user the most important information

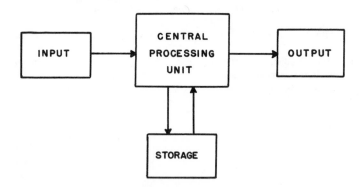

Figure 1. The basic computer hardware configuration.

Table I. List of Inputs and Outputs

Inputs	Outputs
Keyboard	Monitor
Numeric pad	Printer
Joystick	Plotter
Paddle	Speech synthesizer
Graphics tablet or pad	Analog-to-digital converter
Voice analyzer	
Touch-sensitive screen	
Light pen	
Special switch	
Analog-to-digital converter	

quickly and efficiently. The reader should understand, however, that using computers effectively is, in part, dependent on how much the user knows about existing hardware. Staying current on hardware will be a continuing need for the serious user.

INPUTS

Table I contains a list of inputs and outputs. Inputs take information from the outside world and transduce it into electrical codes that the computer can manipulate.

The Keyboard

The most common of the input devices is the keyboard. The keyboard (Fig. 2) has the same letter and number layout as the typewriter. However, there are several special function keys which enhance the capability of the computer. Not all computers have the same special function keys, and only the more widely used ones will be discussed here.

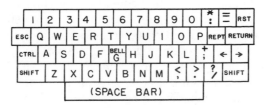

Figure 2. An example of a computer keyboard. ESC, escape; CTRL, control; RST, reset; REPT, repeat.

The control key can be considered a second shift key. By pressing the control key and another key simultaneously, a unique code is input to the computer. Thus, the control key increases the number of available codes that can be input to the computer by as many keys as there are on the keyboard. The escape key is so named because it is often used to "escape" from a program in progress. In reality it is just another key that inputs a unique code. The reset key inputs a code that causes some programs to terminate. Accidentally pressing it while a program is in progress may cause a loss of data. Some computers protect against accidentally pressing the reset key by placing it away from the keyboard or by requiring that a second key be pressed simultaneously.

The return (enter) key on a computer keyboard does not serve the same function as the return key on a typewriter. As you type on a conventional typewriter, the letters print with each key pressed. When working on a computer, the letters appear on the screen as you press them, but they are not input to the computer until the return (enter) key is pressed. Until the return (enter) key is pressed, the input is stored in a *buffer*. When the return (enter) key is pressed, all of the input in the buffer is "dumped" into the computer.

The code that is input to the computer from the keyboard is called ASCII (American Standard Code for Information Interchange). This is one of the few features of computers that is standardized. It was originally developed as the code used by teletype machines to transmit information.

Many keyboards also have separate numeric pads to input numbers more efficiently, and many have several additional function keys, some which the operator can program to use as desired. One of the first things the owner of a new computer should do is to read the manual(s) carefully to determine the capability of the keyboard.

Joysticks, Paddles, and Other Fun Devices

One of the first commercially attractive features of the microcomputer was that it could be used to play games. Video arcades paved the way for home entertainment games that could be programmed to be of almost unlimited complexity. Since inputs from the arcades were of the nature of joysticks and paddles, input ports were also built into personal microcomputers to accommodate these devices. This has been an exceptional benefit in programming for the handicapped because special devices that require only a single switch can be programmed through that input port. This means that the computer can be made to complete any function of which it is capable by a person who can operate a single switch. The benefits to the severely handicapped are far reaching because of this development.

Graphics tablets, many of which have excellent capabilities at a modest cost, are also connected to the computer through the joystick input port. These allow even the unsophisticated user to design high-quality, individualized graphics.

Special Purpose Inputs

Many microcomputers have the capability of being *interfaced,* that is, connected to other devices in such a manner that the microcomputer and the other device can communicate. These microcomputers have *slots,* which are places where special input devices can be connected. Such items as light pens, voice analyzers, and touch-sensitive screens can be used as inputs to the microcomputer. These devices are made to react to some change in the environment, such as pressure, light, or sound, and to enter that change to the computer.

The implications of this capability for the handicapped are staggering. In essence, the computer can be configured to have a receptor system that can be sensitive to the same types of stimuli that activate human receptor systems. The computer can, in effect, be made to "hear," "see," and "feel" things in the environment. One of the obvious possibilities is the use of the computer to compensate for a disordered sensory system. We will spend more time discussing this issue in the chapter on clinical uses.

CENTRAL PROCESSING UNIT

The core of the microcomputer can be found on one IC (integrated circuit) chip. All of the other chips are involved in transmitting information to or from the microprocessor, displaying information, and storing information. The central processing unit (CPU) accepts information from the input devices, manipulates the information as it has been programmed to, and outputs the results to some type of display (screen, printer, plotter, etc.).

The central processing unit can do arithmetic operations (add, subtract, multiply, divide) and perform logical operations on data. Logical operations that can be performed are in the form of conditional statements; e.g., if condition A is present, perform operation B.

Several IC chip processors are commonly used. The 6502 and derivatives of the 6502 are used in Apple and Apple-compatible computers. The Z80, 8080, and their descendants form the basis for CP/M (control program for microcomputer) computers. These microprocessors, which were the first generation, are called *eight-bit machines* because they process data in "chunks" of eight bits. The chunks of bits are called *bytes*. Each bit in the byte is electronically represented by a 0 or 1, and since the bits represent only two states (0 or 1), they operate under the rules of binary math. More will be written on binary math in Chapter 3. Suffice it to say at this point that the computer reads bits as 0 or 1, thus an eight-bit machine can communicate numbers of up to 256 (2 to the eight power). The next generation of microprocessors were 16-bit and the most current is the 32-bit microprocessor (IC chip 68000).

The primary difference between the 8-, 16-, and 32-bit processors is speed. Information that is being processed at 32 bits per second will be processed more quickly. While the number of bits per byte relates to the efficiency of the machine, it does not enhance its capabilities to manipulate data. The 8-bit machine can do all of the operations that the 32-bit machine can do.

In addition to the microprocessor chips, the main chips on the motherboard are the ROM and RAM chips. ROM chips (read-only memory) have programs stored on them that cannot be changed. These allow the computer to do many operations without requiring that special disk programs be loaded. The autostart program is a good example. When the machine is turned on, a program in ROM is initiated to get the user started.

ROM programs are growing in popularity. There are computers now that have the word processing, spreadsheet, and database programs built into the ROM chips so they are immediately available to the user and require no external software.

RAM (random access memory) chips can store information that is put into the computer. The amount of information that can be stored in the computer at one time is dependent on the amount of RAM available. In early models, a RAM chip stored only 1K (kilobyte = 1000 bytes) or 2K of information. It is expected that one of the major breakthroughs in the near future will be the development of RAM chips that can hold megabytes of information.

The importance of large memory is important. In a 64K machine, only about 15–20 pages of text can be processed at one time. When the machine's memory is exhausted, the user has to store the information in the computer at that time in an external device before processing new information. This can be time consuming and inconvenient for word processing and data management. In addition, software that deals in sophisticated logic, such as AI (artificial intelligence), may need considerably more dynamic memory than most microcomputers now have. One of the major obstacles to overcome in creating computers that can simulate the human thought process is dynamic memory. That obstacle will most likely be removed in the next few years.

Other chips in the computer act as "gates" to move information electronically from one component of the computer to another or from the computer to external devices.

OUTPUTS

When the data that have been input to the microprocessor are analyzed, the results of that analysis must be output if the operator is to know the results. Results stored in a computer are meaningless if they cannot be seen. The most common output device is a monitor.

Monitors

Monitors are screens on which patterns of light can be displayed. Many computers have adapters that allow them to use a television screen as a monitor. Monitor screens may be monochrome (green on black, amber on black) or color. The key characteristics of screens of which the user needs to be aware are color and resolution. If the user has software that displays results in color, the full potential of the programs can be appreciated only in color. However, programs written for color can be displayed on monochrome screens, with the different colors registering as different shades. The effect, unfortunately, falls short of desirable.

Programs not written to use color (such as word processing software) can be displayed on any type of monitor. However, the resolution (clarity of display) for monochrome programs is better on a monochrome monitor. Color monitors tend to add tints of color to script and thus are not practical for a person doing a lot of word/data processing. (In effect, this means the user who must do both word processing and use programs in which color is important should have two monitors: one color and one monochrome).

Resolution is also related to the number of dots (pixels) that can be lighted on the screen. The greater the number of pixels, the more desirable the image. As might be expected, monitors with greater numbers of pixels are more expensive. The resolution is most important when using programs that utilize graphics.

Color monitors are divided into two general classes: composite and RGB (red, green, blue). The composite monitor utilizes one line for input whereas the RGB monitor splits the signal into three components. Because of this, the RGB monitors provide higher resolution and are more desirable for programs utilizing color graphics. Again, as expected, the RGB monitors are more costly.

Careful consideration should be given to the choice of a monitor since it will be used each time the computer is turned on. The eye comfort and ease of reading will have far-reaching effects in the long-run usage of the system.

Printers

In almost all operations there is a need for a *hard copy,* or a permanent copy of the text or program on paper. For this reason, most people would not consider a system complete without a printer.

There are basically two kinds of printers. One type prints in exactly the same manner as a typewriter; that is, an image of the letter strikes against a ribbon to leave an imprint on paper. The second type is called *dot matrix.* This type of printer lays out a pattern of small dots that collectively make up the outline of each printed letter. The dots are imprinted on the paper by the ends of wires in the printhead. A vertical line of seven or more wires in the print head makes it possible to print any letter configuration imaginable. For this reason, dot matrix printers can be used to print in more than one language with no physical modification. Figure 3 demonstrates how dots are laid out in patterns to form letters.

Dot matrix printers are less expensive and print at a much higher rate of speed than typewriter-like printers. However, the quality of print is not as good. *Letter-quality* printers are ones that print an image that is comparable to that of an office-quality typewriter. Some dot matrix printers can lay out patterns that are sharper by overlapping dots. While they are close to letter quality, they still lack the sharp image of the letter-quality printer. These models of dot matrix printers are said to have correspondence quality since the quality is acceptable for most forms of correspond-

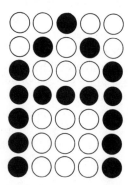

Figure 3. How characters are made from dot matrix: shown here is the letter *A*.

ence. When working in correspondence mode, dot matrix printers sacrifice speed for quality.

A typical dot matrix printer can print at a speed of 160 cps (characters per second) in normal mode and 40 cps in correspondence-quality mode. The letter quality printers can print at about 20 cps. This means that in a normal situation a double-spaced page (33 lines, 60 characters per line) would require the following amounts of time to be printed:

Dot matrix—normal mode	12 seconds
Dot matrix—correspondence mode	50 seconds
Letter quality	99 seconds

A 10-page manuscript would require

Dot matrix—normal mode	2 minutes
Dot matrix—correspondence mode	8 + minutes
Letter quality	16½ minutes

If the user has a large volume of material to print, the time saved in using a dot matrix is substantial. However, if quality is the main consideration, then there is no substitute for the letter-quality printer.

It should also be noted that printers can be noisy. A consideration in choosing a printer should be the noise output level and available accessories that can reduce noise (noise-buffering covers, pads to set the printer on, etc.).

A comparison of the print types and quality of print is shown in Fig. 4.

With the appropriate interface hardware, dot matrix printers can print graphics on paper. This is accomplished by putting dots or other shapes in configurations to reflect shading patterns of pictures. Examples of computer-generated graphics are shown in Fig. 5.

The user should also look at such things as buffer size, feed mechanism, and ribbon. The *buffer size* determines how much information can be "dumped" from the computer to the printer at one time. Since the computer dumps information much faster than the printer can print it, a small buffer means that the computer has to wait for the printer to catch up. A larger buffer can allow several pages to be dumped from the computer to the printer at one time, thereby leaving the computer free for the user to go on to the next task. Buffer sizes for printers usually range from 1K to 16K. For the most efficient operation, a larger buffer size is needed.

The feed mechanism is also important to consider. "Computer paper" is so designated because it is a chain of paper with holes along either side which allows the paper to be pulled through by cogs, or *pins*. This type

REGULAR DOT MATRIX

```
"#$%&'()*+,-./0123456789:;<=>?@ABCDEFGHIJKLMNOPQRSTUVWXYZ[\]^_`abcdefghijklmnopq
#$%&'()*+,-./0123456789:;<=>?@ABCDEFGHIJKLMNOPQRSTUVWXYZ[\]^_`abcdefghijklmnopqr
$%&'()*+,-./0123456789:;<=>?@ABCDEFGHIJKLMNOPQRSTUVWXYZ[\]^_`abcdefghijklmnopqrs
%&'()*+,-./0123456789:;<=>?@ABCDEFGHIJKLMNOPQRSTUVWXYZ[\]^_`abcdefghijklmnopqrst
```

CORRESPONDENCE QUALITY

```
"#$%&'()*+,-./0123456789:;<=>?@ABCDEFGHIJKLMNOPQRSTUVWXYZ[\]^_`abcdefghijklmnopq
#$%&'()*+,-./0123456789:;<=>?@ABCDEFGHIJKLMNOPQRSTUVWXYZ[\]^_`abcdefghijklmnopqr
$%&'()*+,-./0123456789:;<=>?@ABCDEFGHIJKLMNOPQRSTUVWXYZ[\]^_`abcdefghijklmnopqrs
%&'()*+,-./0123456789:;<=>?@ABCDEFGHIJKLMNOPQRSTUVWXYZ[\]^_`abcdefghijklmnopqrst
```

LETTER QUALITY

```
"#$%&'()*+,-./0123456789:;<=>?@ABCDEFGHIJKLMNOPQRSTUVWXYZ[\]^_`abcdefghijklmnopq
#$%&'()*+,-./0123456789:;<=>?@ABCDEFGHIJKLMNOPQRSTUVWXYZ[\]^_`abcdefghijklmnopqr
$%&'()*+,-./0123456789:;<=>?@ABCDEFGHIJKLMNOPQRSTUVWXYZ[\]^_`abcdefghijklmnopqrs
%&'()*+,-./0123456789:;<=>?@ABCDEFGHIJKLMNOPQRSTUVWXYZ[\]^_`abcdefghijklmnopqrst
```

Figure 4. A comparison of print quality for standard dot matrix, correspondence quality, and letter quality print.

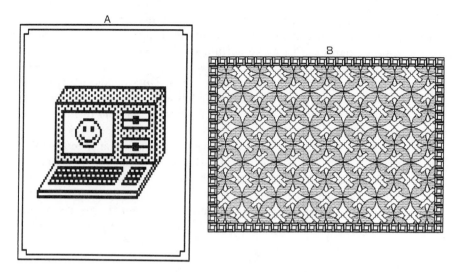

Figure 5. Examples of computer-generated graphics.

of feed mechanism is called *tractor* or *pin* feed and is necessary if the user is going to use computer paper. The second type of mechanism is called *friction* feed. This is the same type of feed mechanism that you find on a typewriter, and it can be used with any type of paper. So, if letterhead stationery is going to be used, a friction feed is necessary. The obvious choice is to buy a printer that has both. Having only one or the other would limit the range of uses of the computer severely.

Ribbons play a small role in the overall operation, but buying and changing them can be a major problem. There is no industry standard for printer ribbons. Some use regular typewriter ribbons and others have fairly complex mechanisms. Before buying a printer, find out how much the ribbon costs and then change one to determine how easy or difficult it is. Most printers have quickly changed, snap-in, snap-out ribbon cartridges. While these ribbons may cost slightly more, the ease of use is probably worth the price differential.

Printers receive information from the computer through either a serial or parallel output. A printer that is configured for accepting information from a parallel output cannot work with a serial output and vice versa.

Serial outputs transmit information one bit of information at a time. Parallel outputs transmit several bits (one byte) of information simultaneously and therefore have a faster transmission rate. Serial outputs may have more versatility because they can be used with other peripheral devices, such as modems for telephone transmission. Buyers should realize that a printer requires an interface to the computer and sometimes the interface is not an integral part of the computer or printer package. Check at the time of purchase to make certain that the right interface for the printer is included.

Another type of printer is based on ink jets. Dots of ink are sprayed onto the paper to configure matrices for characters as described before. These printers have the advantages of being quiet, fast, and forming very good quality print.

Laser printers can produce excellent print at phenomenal speed. At the present time the cost of laser printers is prohibitive, but this is expected to change in the near future. Laser printers can produce book-length manuscripts in a matter of minutes.

The best way to determine which printer will meet the user's needs best is to see them and compare price, quality, and ease of use.

Plotters

Plotters are output devices that can produce line drawings, bar graphs, pie charts, and other such representations of data in color. Plotters can have any number of colors, but the most common arrangement is a four-color plotter. The plotter works on the basis of colored pens moving on a mechanical arm. The movement of the mechanism is two dimensional; that is, it can plot an X, Y axis. Plotters can produce statistics displays, such as bar graphs, line graphs, or pie charts. Plotters are also used extensively with CAD (computer-assisted design) software packages.

While a plotter is not considered a standard component in a basic microcomputer setup, it would warrant consideration if graphic representation of data is important. Speed, reliability, and ease of use are key characteristics to consider in choosing one.

Speech Analyzers

Since the field of communication disorders deals with human communication, devices that recognize and produce voice are desirable for many applications. Both types of devices work on the principle of manipulating an analog signal (an analog signal is one that is constantly changing).

Voice analyzers accept the signal through a microphone. A special interface card that plugs into the computer is needed to convert the analog signal to digital information which the computer can store. In the most basic type of analysis (analog to digital) the voice analyzer samples the voltage of the incoming signal at discrete time intervals and stores that voltage in the computer. Figure 6 is a graphic representation of the process. More discrete analysis is achieved by increasing the sample rate (decreasing the time interval between samples) so that a more complete picture of the signal is stored.

The basic analog-to-digital (A/D) process has the drawback of producing amounts of information that require large-scale storage capacity. For example, to achieve a truly accurate picture of a speech signal, the sample rate needs to be 20,000 samples per second. Each sample must be stored in a cell, so the computer must have 20,000 cells devoted to storing the sample. A microcomputer with 128K capacity could store only 6 seconds (actually less because part of the memory would be used to store the analyzing program). A/D converters will be discussed more fully later in Chapter 8.

Analysis techniques are now being developed that use less memory through selective sampling. In effect, the computer is programmed to identify salient characteristics of the signal and store that information only.

Speech Synthesizers

Synthesis techniques mirror analysis techniques. Voice can be reproduced from a stored sample by outputting the stored voltage values in the same sequence in which they were input. The result is an analog signal that drives a speaker, creating sound that is reflective of input. This is called *digitally encoded speech.*

Another type of synthesized speech is produced by phoneme splicing. Analog signals for individual phonemes of the language are stored and the user selects the phonemes in the sequence that are desired. This type of synthesis results in an output which is monotone and easily identified by

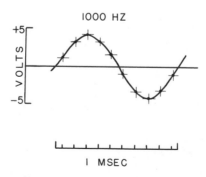

Figure 6.   A demonstration of the basis for analog-to-digital signal conversion.

the listener as produced by a computer (computer speech). Prosodic features such as pitch and intensify contours are often missing. In addition the transitional elements of the acoustic signal which provide contiguity from one phoneme to the next are lacking. The technology is improving rapidly in this area, however, and in the near future we may see machines that challenge the listener to determine whether or not they are human or machine.

STORAGE DEVICES

Dynamic Memory (RAM)

Memory within the machine itself (random access memory, or RAM) is found on IC chips. RAM was discussed briefly earlier in this chapter under "Central Processing Unit." The amount of memory is stated in terms of kilobytes (K). The first truly functional microcomputers had 48K. As technology improved the capacity of chips for storage, this climbed to 64K, 128K, and extensions beyond this. In functional terms, each byte contains a specified number of bits. The first microcomputers were 8-bit machines, the next generation 16-bit, and then 32-bit, again with the capacity improving as technology improves. Because microcomputers move information in bytes (several bits at a time), the more bits per byte, the faster the machine processes information and the more storage capacity per kilobyte.

The information stored on the RAM chips in the machine is referred to as *dynamic memory*. Dynamic memory is instantaneously available for processing; however, the information stored on the RAM chips is lost whenever the power to the machine is turned off. The greater the memory of the machine, the more information that can be held for processing at any one time. The machine with a larger memory has obvious advantages for activities requiring large databases or other substantial amounts of information which need to be processed at one time.

Passive Memory

Devices external to the microcomputer that store information include cassettes, floppy disks, and hard disks. On computer cassettes, like the kind used with audio recordings, the information is electronically encoded on the tape. Cassettes have the disadvantage of slow speed; the need to rewind, and when there is more than one thing stored on the cassette, the need to locate information, can be a time-consuming chore.

Floppy disks and hard disks can store and access information more quickly. Both have information electronically encoded in the same manner as the cassette. The floppy disk is descriptively named. It is flexible, and composed of basically the same material as the cassette tape, only packaged on a circular diskette. The diskette is stored in a static-free cover that protects it from the environment. The only part of the diskette that is exposed is the part needed for accessing data. Information is communicated through a head (in the same manner as a cassette recorder) inside the disk drive. Storage capacity is usually measured in terms of kilobytes (K).

Floppy disks are reliable. They will last about as long as an audio cassette tape. The main dangers in damaging a disk come from spilling fluids on it (the rule should be, no coffee near the computer area), bending it (do not lay heavy objects on it or store it in a bent position), and setting it near magnetic fields (do not set it on the monitor, disk drives, computer, or any other devices that generate electrical fields). Even small permanent magnets, such as the ones found in desk-top paper clip holders, can cause damage.

Hard disks are made of metal alloys. Because the material that the disk is made of is more dense, more data can be stored electronically. Hard disk storage is usually stated in terms of megabytes (millions of bytes; M) of information. Hard disks are generally encased in protective covers to prevent environmental damage. They are more reliable than floppy disks for long-term storage of information.

DISK OPERATING SYSTEMS

Unfortunately, getting information to and from disks can be a bit more complicated than it sounds. First of all, there are several different disk operating systems (DOS). The DOS is the internal code which allows a computer to communicate with a storage device. A new disk is blank when purchased. Before information can be communicated to the disk, the computer has to place an operating system on the disk. The process of encoding an operating system on a disk is called *initialization*. This has two effects worth noting. One, part of the space on the disk used for storing information is reserved for the DOS. Two, disks can only be accessed if the operating system of the computer with which the user is trying to access it is compatible with the operating system of the computer which initialized the disk originally. In effect, this means that an Apple computer cannot access a disk initialized by a CP/M computer or an IBM PC computer.

If an agency is considering purchasing more than one computer, the compatibility of the disk operating systems should be a consideration, if the agency wants to be able to use the disks created on one computer with the others.

MODEMS

Modems (modulator–demodulator) are devices that allow computers to communicate across conventional telephone lines. There is an increasing utilization of modems to link personal computers (the term *personal computer* is used interchangeably with *microcomputer*) and with larger computers.

Modem capability is built into some microcomputers while others require additional equipment. Some modems connect directly through the phone lines (from computer to the phone jack) and others connect to the handset (these are called *acoustic modems*). Probably the most significant aspect of a modem to consider is the rate at which it can transmit and receive information. Rates are stated in *baud* (bits per second). Although baud rates between 110 and 9600 are possible, 300 baud and 1200 baud are the most common rates for transmitting information from computer to computer at the present time. However, faster baud rates are expected to become more commonplace in the near future. Faster baud rates are preferred because information is transmitted more rapidly and less telephone time is required. As is usually the case, the higher the baud rate, the more costly is the piece of equipment. Access charges for commercial databases are also often more costly for modems with higher baud rates.

Other features which modems may have include automatic dialing or answering (regardless of the presence of the user), time displays (to indicate how long the connection has been made—this could have an impact on telephone bills), and automatic disconnect (to "hang up" at a predetermined condition). It is generally desirable to have all of the features listed above if the user plans to make extensive use of the modem.

Modems must have software that will provide the user with control over the transmission process. The ease of use of software (and ensuring that the software is included as part of the modem package) should be investigated before purchase. The prospective user should be aware that many modems DO NOT have their own software. For those modems, software must be purchased separately or written especially for them.

THE FUTURE IN HARDWARE

The fast-paced developments in technology to this point suggest that the future may provide even more uses than we can now conceptualize.

One thing is for certain: if the behavioral sciences fields, such as communication disorders, are to keep pace with the technology, the members must stay abreast of developments and create hardware and software systems that will open the door for full use of the potential of the machine.

References

Ahl, D. (1983). Buying a printer. *Creative Computing, 9,* 12–29.

Anderson, J. (1983). Print about printers. *Creative Computing, 9,* 30–61.

Bonner, P., & Keogh, J. (1984). Connected! A buyer's guide on modems. *Personal Computing, 8,* 146–152, 195.

Boraiko, A. (1982). The chip. *National Geographic, 162,* 421–476.

Edelson, R. (1984). Characters per second: A guide to selecting the perfect printer. *Interface Age,* June, 59–63, 128–138.

Gabel, D. (1983). Printing á la mode. *Personal Computing, 7,* 116–123.

Keogh, J. (1983). The perfect peripheral for the working computer. *Personal Computing, 7,* 64–77, 214–215.

Miller, D. (1983). Videotex: Science fiction or reality? *Byte, 8,* 42–56.

Osgood, D. (1985). The KoalaPad. *Byte, 10,* 283–286.

Powell, B. (1984). Monitors. *Popular Computing, 3,* 122–135.

Sehr, R. (1984). How hard disks can save you time as well as space. *Personal Computing, 8,* 152–160.

Townsley, D., & Venning-Townsley, F. (1984). Monitors in monochrome. *A +, 2,* 60–67.

Walker, L. (1984). A complete buyer's guide to monitors. *Personal Computing, 8,* 194–205.

Young, J. (1984). How to paint with your computer. *Personal Computing, 8,* 126–137.

3

Software

The mystique of "computing" has led many persons to believe that the computer is a self-perpetuating form of intelligence that can do anything. Nothing is further from the truth. The computer by itself has no value and is only as useful as the tasks for which it is programmed. The computer belongs in the same "tool box" as the typewriter, calculator, and copier. By itself it is a chunk of conductors, insulators, and semiconductors that occupies space. Only through application does it have value.

The computer is passive. It does not generate any form of interchange with the environment by itself. Like a mindless slave, it does everything it is told and like a mindless slave, it must be told what to do in very specific terms. That is the purpose of software. Software is the set of instructions which directs the computer to perform desired actions.

Since the computer is only as good as the software written for it, it is important to understand how software works. To do this, we need to understand how the computer processes instructions.

OF BYTES AND BITS

The basic unit of processing is the *bit*. This is a single piece of information which is encoded electrically as one of two states. In one state, there is an electrical charge present. This is usually graphically coded as *1* (one). In the other state, there is no electrical charge present, usually coded graphically as *0* (zero). The entire operation of the computer is based on processing information that is encoded in these two states—an exceptionally limited symbol system.

However, properly utilized, the computer can translate bits into information and a variety of operations. Much of the operation is based on binary mathematics, so we will take some time to discuss it at this point.

Turning Bits into Action

Binary mathematics has the same operations as the decimal system. For example, there are the columns for the "ones," "tens," "hundreds," and so on, as indicated below. However, "ten," "hundred," and the rest of the places have different values in binary and in decimal systems. Since we have only two symbols, addition works in the following manner:

$$
\begin{array}{r}
1 \\
+1 \\
\hline
10
\end{array}
$$

Because there is no higher symbol in binary mathematics than 1, we put a 0 in the ones column and carry the 1 to the tens column. An example of binary and decimal mathematics is shown below.

Binary	Decimal

$$
\begin{array}{rr}
1 & 1 \\
+1 & +1 \\
\hline
10 & 2
\end{array}
$$

$$
\begin{array}{rr}
10 & 2 \\
+10 & +2 \\
\hline
100 & 4
\end{array}
$$

$$
\begin{array}{rr}
100 & 4 \\
+100 & +4 \\
\hline
1000 & 8
\end{array}
$$

Carrying this further, we find the following binary numbers and decimal equivalents:

Binary	Decimal
1	1
10	2
11	3
100	4
101	5
110	6
111	7
1000	8
1001	9
1010	10
10000	16
100000	32
1000000	64
10000000	128
100000000	256

For humans, the greater numbers of symbols involved in binary coding poses the problem of too many symbols to process at one time. However, the computer works at extraordinary speeds with near-perfect accuracy so the binary system works very well for it. And fortunately for us, the computer has been constructed in such a way that it accepts decimal values and does the binary coding itself, thereby relieving us of having to make the conversion.

After values are input to the computer, the computer manipulates them in the manner desired by the user. The computer has built-in functions, or manipulations it can perform on the data. These include arithmetic functions (addition, subtraction, multiplication, division, squaring the number, etc.) and logic functions. Logic functions include comparative capabilities which result in a decision being made. Decisions can be made on the basis of several criteria. We will discuss these processes more fully in the following section on languages.

Computer Languages

When computers were first made it was recognized that they would have very limited potential if users had to code information in a binary format. Early computer developers established hardware and software to overcome that problem. First, rather than forcing the user to code information, the computer was interfaced (connected with) a keyboard with standard symbols (i.e., numbers, letters, and other symbols). This keyboard was built so that when a key was struck, a binary number was input to the computer. That binary number is generated from a special chip which translates input from specific keys on the keyboard into a binary equivalent. The computer is designed to differentiate these symbols on the basis of the binary coding. For example, *A* is coded as the binary number 1000001 (decimal 65), *B* is 1000010 (decimal 66), *C* is 1000011 (decimal 67), and so on. This code is known as ASCII (American Standard Code for Information Interchange) and is the industry standard for keyboards.

Designers took the concept of computer recognition of code a step further and built into the computer the ability to recognize sequences of symbols and interpret those sequences as instructions. This, of course, is the same form of communication used between humans, so the encoding process was called a *language*. Several different computer languages have been developed; some have become widespread and others are used only by specialized groups of programmers.

The most common language used in programming in general is BASIC (Beginners All-purpose Symbolic Instruction Code), which was developed at Dartmouth in 1951. BASIC is also the language most widely used at the present time in programming diagnosis and treatment programs in communicative disorders. BASIC is relatively easy to learn, allows a great deal of versatility in programming, and has commands similar to English. It is also a computer language that is well suited for dealing with words. Early program languages such as FORTRAN and COBOL were well suited to the fields in which they were applied (FORTRAN in fields closely allied to mathematics, COBOL in business), but were oriented to handle numbers more efficiently than words.

Because of its versatility and widespread application, BASIC will be the language used to discuss examples of concepts of computer programming in this chapter. It should be understood, however, that the language used does not change how the computer works. Different languages are simply different codes which permit the user to enter information and instructions into the computer. Computers work the same, regardless of the language used to program them.

BASIC Examples

Let us look at how the computer handles a simple math problem. The following program (written in BASIC) will add two numbers.

```
10   INPUT A
20   INPUT B
30   C = A + B
40   PRINT C
```

This program works as follows. First, the instructions are carried out in ascending order of the line numbers. Line 10 prints a question mark on the screen and tells the computer to look for an input from the keyboard. Nothing else will occur until a number is typed and the return key pressed. When the number is typed and return pressed, the computer stores the number that is input as a variable with the name A.

Then the program moves to line 20, which like line 10 tells the computer to wait for a number to be typed and the return key pressed. When this is done, the number that was typed is stored as a variable with the name B. Line 30 adds the value of A and B and stores that value as C. Notice that variables are defined on the left side of the equals sign.

If we stopped at this point, the computer will have added the numbers, but we would not know the answer. To see the answer, we have to tell the computer to print the value of variable C. Line 40 accomplishes this.

Obviously, to write a program that would perform the operation only one time would be foolish. It would take more time to write than to add the numbers by using a calculator. The value of such a program is that it can be run time and time again and the answer will be computed accurately and instantly when the variables are changed in response to the input prompts. In an example such as the above, the program would have little value over using a simple hand calculator. To add two one-digit numbers would require four keystrokes (three keystrokes on some) on a hand calculator and four keystrokes on a computer. Obviously there is no saving gained using the computer with simple addition. However, if the calculation on line 30 was more complex, such as

    30   $C = A*(B + A/B)/(B/A)$

the computer would be considerably more efficient. The computer would still only require four keystrokes for this problem while the calculator would require about 15. The more complex and lengthy the calculation, the more valuable the computer to the computation process.

Logical Processes

In addition to being able to manipulate numbers with speed and precision, the computer can be programmed to follow a path of logic. The principal logic operation is the IF . . . THEN statement. The IF . . . THEN statement allows the computer to compare two pieces of information and make a decision based on the relationship of those two pieces of information. The following example is from an 11-year-old who attended one of the author's computer camps.

```
10  HOME:VTAB10
20  INPUT "HOW OLD ARE YOU? " ;X
30  IF X>15 THEN 50
40  PRINT:PRINT:PRINT "THAT'S A GOOD AGE!":END
50  PRINT:PRINT:PRINT "BOY! THAT'S OLD!":END
```

The first line tells the computer to clear the screen and put the cursor down 10 lines on the screen. Line 20 requests input from the user in response to the prompt "HOW OLD ARE YOU?" Line 30 is the decision-making operation. If X (which stands for whatever number was input by the user) is greater than 15, the program jumps to line 50 and prints "BOY! THAT'S OLD!" If X is not greater than 15, then it goes on to the next statement, which tells the computer to print "THAT'S A GOOD AGE!"

Most computer programs rely heavily on conditional statements. For example, most programs have menus which are numbered (or lettered) as follows:

```
WHICH DO YOU WANT:
  1. CONTINUE
  2. RETURN TO BEGINNING
  3. TERMINATE PROGRAM
```

When the user inputs the number, the computer processes it through the conditional statement and proceeds to the line of the program to which it was directed. The computer can also compare other characters, such as in the case of a screen prompt which reads

```
DO YOU WANT TO CONTINUE? (Y/N)
```

The computer compares the letter input and proceeds to the next step directed. The actual program might look like this:

```
4000  INPUT "DO YOU WANT TO CONTINUE? (Y/N) ";X$
4010  IF X$="Y" THEN 4040
4020  IF X$<>"N" THEN 4000
4030  END
4040  (more program statements)
```

Line 4000 asks the user to enter something in response to DO YOU WANT TO CONTINUE? (Y/N). If the user enters Y then control goes to statement 4040 and the program continues. If the user enters N, the computer checks through statements 4010 and 4020 and terminates the program. Line 4020 is an *error-trapping* routine. If for some reason the user strikes a key other than Y or N, program control will branch to line 4000 and the request for input will be repeated.

Learning to program is not particularly difficult, but it is time consuming. The reader who would like to learn more about programming is referred to the list of references at the end of this chapter. For the individual who would like the experience of keying in some simple BASIC programs, Appendix A contains some utility programs that might be of use in a clinical setting. Some of these will be discussed in later chapters.

SOFTWARE DEVELOPMENT

One of the first facts of life that is learned in working with computers is the cost of software. It is awe-inspiring to consider that a few $3 diskettes with a program on them and an instruction manual on how to operate the program may cost several hundred dollars. Certainly the cost is not in reproducing the diskettes, as they can be produced quickly and inexpensively.

Software Worth

The reason for the cost is found in free enterprise. If a program can do something more efficiently than had been done previously, and if there is a need for doing that something more efficiently, then people will pay the price. Many programs that cost hundreds of dollars will pay for themselves in a very short time through the time savings that they afford. There is no area in business in which the law of supply and demand is more actively applied than in the business of producing software.

Deciding whether to buy a piece of software should not be based on the price so much as on the value the software has for the user. For example, one might find a very attractive mathematics tutorial program for $19.95. However, if the user has no need for a mathematics tutorial, then the program is not worth the price. On the other hand, if a piece of software can save the user an average of 2 hours per week on report writing, it can cost several hundred dollars and still be worth it. Two hours per week of time multiplied by 52 weeks per year results in a savings of over 100 hours for the first years alone, a savings of over 2 weeks in manhours.

Software developers also invest much time and effort in the construction of a program. Programs generally start as ideas on how to do something more easily, quickly, accurately, or efficiently. The first step in translating the idea into a functional program is to develop algorithms. An algorithm is a detailed list of steps to be followed in the resolution of a problem.

The algorithm then has to be translated into instructions that the computer can understand. Because the computer has a finite amount of storage and a limited number of operations it can perform, the steps of the algorithm must be made to conform to the constraints of the computer and the computer language used. While learning a programming language is not particularly difficult, developing a useful piece of software that is easy to use and does exactly what it is supposed to do can be quite a challenge.

For an idea to be *programmable* it must be of a nature that permits reaching a conclusion based on logic. Not all processes (especially those generated by human thinking) are based on logic. Processes that require insight are probably beyond the scope of computer programming, unless the "insight" process can be reduced to a number of logical steps.

Polishing the Program

After all of the above conditions have been met, the programmer writes the program. Then he begins what many programmers feel is the most difficult part, which is debugging the program and revising it to make it do the job better. The programmer does much of the debugging by sitting at the keyboard and actually trying different things in running the program to see how they work. Getting the language errors corrected is no great challenge, but finding logic errors and correcting them can be difficult and time consuming.

The developer's goal is to produce a piece of software that is easy to use and on which it is hard to make a mistake. To produce such a work, the programmer has to think of all the procedural and keyboarding errors that an individual could make and put in error-trapping routines. These are routines which detect when the individual has input something or done something for which the program was not intended. Computers have built-in error detection protocols that halt the program when an error is identified. This can cause the program to *crash* (come to an end), which not only interrupts the program, but may lose data that the user has input to the computer. However, error detection routines can be programmed into the software. The computer can be programmed to identify the error and, rather than crash when the error is identified, print a statement on the screen which tells the user what error was made and how to correct it.

For example, some routines require that one diskette be removed from the drive and a second inserted. If the user forgets to do this, and tries to continue running the program with the first diskette still in the disk drive, an error-trapping routine should detect that the correct diskette has not been inserted, put a message to that effect on the screen, and give instructions on how to correct the situation. The more error-trapping routines a program contains, the easier it is to use and the less the chances that a program-crashing error will occur.

Field Testing

The most important test for programs designed for communication disorders is how well they work in the field. No matter how technically correct a program is written, it is only as valuable as its application. Field tests are conducted in different ways. Usually the program is sent to several individuals who run it and then fill out an evaluation sheet, suggesting changes. Changes usually take the form of reducing redundant material (either input or output), simplifying procedures, changing the wording of instructions, and adding subroutines that give the computer greater capability.

The software should go back out to the field several times. The author of this text is fortunate in that he has several field sites in which the software that he develops is used regularly. This permits continued observation, and he has found that watching someone else use a program may lead him to make an important change that the user may not have considered requesting (simply because the user did not know that it could be done). Also, it is important to have the programs run repeatedly to make sure that there is not some obscure error. One of the author's programs had been run over 1800 times in field settings before one minor error was identified.

Persevering Programmers

Most programs of any complexity require hundreds of hours of time on the part of the programmer. Writing the program is the easiest, most interesting part. Going back and rewriting, continuing to make the changes needed to make it a more effective program, is the difficult part. Anyone contemplating programming marketable software needs to be aware of the effort and dedication that it takes to produce a good quality product. Most programmers will agree that no matter how long one works on a program, there is always something else that can be done to make it faster, more efficient, easier to use, etc. It is often heard among computer folks that a program is never finished, the programmer just finally quits working on it.

BUILDING THE SOFTWARE LIBRARY

Software consideration should be first in setting the budget. It is relatively easy to determine how much the buyer will have to spend for a basic hardware configuration. Software, however, is open ended. How much you buy will be limited only by your budget. With many good quality hardware systems starting at less than $1000, the buyer will find that it is not long before expenditures for software far exceed those for hardware. Therefore, the buyer should have a planning strategy for software acquisition.

Commercial Software

The first consideration should be for software which will provide the most immediate help to the clinical program. In most cases, this will be word processing and related programs. Word processing programs, which will be discussed more fully in the next chapter, provide the professional with a tool for writing that far exceeds anything to date. It is estimated that the skilled user reduces the paperwork preparation time over 50% from b.c. (before computer) operations. For a busy professional with reports, budgets, and letters to prepare, this represents a substantial savings in time. Professionals should use computers for the word processing power alone, even if they have no other application. The result in time savings far exceeds the investment in time, effort, and money.

Word processing packages can be general or specific in purpose. It is important for the prospective buyer to work with the word processing package long enough to feel comfortable with it before he buys.

Data processing packages, which also will be discussed in the next chapter, provide the user with the capability of preparing reports which require numerical manipulations, such as monthly, quarterly, and yearly reports on caseload, productivity, and financial status. Persons who have worked with spreadsheets realize the time required to make the necessary calculation to balance the sheet, and the time that is required for preparing billings by typewriter is considerable. The computer can reduce the time required to complete the task and produce a hard-copy output that is more professional in appearance.

There are general and specific types of data management software. Word processing can often be integrated with the data management software. The individual who needs to keep track of data and procedure reports for purposes such as accreditation processes, yearly reports, financial transactions, and grants will find data processing to be an excellent toool.

Other than word and data processing software, the type of software purchased is based on specific needs. Software for the diagnosis and treatment of speech and language disorders will be discussed in Chapters 6 and 7. Software for the diagnosis and treatment of hearing disorders will be discussed in Chapters 8 and 9. At this point, however, there are some general guidelines that can be applied to the evaluation of all software.

Software Budgeting

First of all, the budget should be based on specific items. This is especially true for those just initiating programs. The original budget is often considered to be a one-time expenditure. That is, once the initial outlay is made, the agency often is not receptive to further purchases.

Software is now displayed at most conferences of any size. It would be well worth the time and travel expense to go to a regional, or better, national conference and plan to spend a day or two in the exhibit hall trying out software. Some of the conferences include a computer resource room at which there are several types of computers and a large stock of software which can be checked out to be evaluated by the user. This is an ideal way to get acquainted with software and at the same time prepare a software budget.

Software budget planning for the initial program should include the following:

Word processing software	$75—500
Data processing software	$100—700
Utilities programs	$100—500
Communication disorders software	$40—1000 per program

The amount of software that can be purchased for specific clinical or administrative purposes will be determined to some extent by the capability that the user desires in word and data processing.

The prospective buyer should determine the amount of use a program will get, the amount of time/effort that can be saved, and the amount of time/effort needed to learn the program and then weigh those considerations against price. Estimates in this regard should be made on a very practical basis, i.e., by calculating actually how many times during a given period of time a piece of software will be used and how much time will be saved by its use. For example, a piece of software that will be used once a week, and save an hour each time it is used, will save over 1 week in manhours (40+ hours) in a year of use. Price by itself, however, should never be the primary concern.

Software Reviewing Procedures

There have been several reviewing tools developed to provide the user with an approach to assessing software. As Chairman of the ASHA Committee on Educational Technology, the author was involved in the development of such a tool for communicative disorders. It was based on the checklist in Table II. This checklist was modified slightly and adopted

Table II. Software Review Checksheet

Score using the following: 1. Poor 2. Fair 3. Good 4. Excellent 5. Not applicable

1. Program description
   a. Is the purpose of the program clearly defined? —
   b. Is the manner in which the program works clearly described? —
   c. Are the instructions for getting started with the program clearly described? —
   d. Are the instructions for storing and retrieving data clearly described? —
   e. Are hardware requirements clearly stated? —
2. Program effectiveness
   a. Is the software program logical and reasonable? —
   b. Will the program produce consistent results in various settings under various conditions? —
   c. Is there a reprint of an article, a technical report, or other information describing the results of a study(ies) of effectiveness? —
3. User friendliness
   a. Is the program easy to enter, e.g., a turnkey system? —
   b. Is the program easy to exit? —
   c. Are the instructions displayed on the screen easy to understand and complete? —
   d. Are the input responses to the machine familiar (such as Y for yes and N for no)? —
   e. Are program options displayed as "menus"? —
   f. What does the program do if the user strikes a wrong key (does it give a prompt reminding him of the correct options and disregard the error)? —
   g. Can input errors be easily corrected? —
   h. Are data outputs easily retrieved? —
   j. Are data outputs complete and attractively formatted? —
4. Support/documentation
   a. Is the documentation complete (does it tell you everything you need to know)? —
   b. Is the documentation concise (does it tell you *more* than you want to know)? —
   c. Is the documentation written in terms you can understand? —
   d. Is the documentation well organized (can you find answers to specific problems by referring to an index or table of contents)? —
   e. Does it adequately describe the hardware needed and any special instruction for its use? —
   f. Are hardware and software options clearly explained? —
   g. Is there a source for help (someone to call or write if you have a question)? —
   h. Are backup copies provided (if not, are instructions for making backup copies included)? —
   j. Can the program be returned if the user decides that it is not appropriate for his setting? —
   k. Can replacement copies be obtained at a reduced rate if the originals become damaged? —
   l. Can updated program revisions be obtained at a reduced rate? —

Summary of ratings[a]
   1. Program description —
   2. Program effectiveness —
   3. User friendliness —
   4. Support/documentation —
   5. Overall rating[b] —

[a]Summaries of ratings are the averages of items in each category.
[b]The overall rating may be different from the average of the summary ratings.

as the protocol for reviewing software for the Materials Section of the *Asha* journal (American Speech–Language–Hearing Association, 1984) and the *Journal of Computer Users in Speech and Hearing* (Fitch, 1985). The formal reviews of new software by professionals in the field found in these journals can be an excellent resource for staying current on software developments. However, regardless of the professional reviews, individual users should make final considerations only after their own review of the material.

The most important review will be that done in your own setting. It is recommended that each new program be evaluated according to the criteria in Table II before purchase. Legitimate, respectable companies will permit the prospective buyer time to review the software before making a firm decision. This may take the form of a trial review period during which the program can be returned if found not to be appropriate. Some companies will have sample, or tutorial, programs available. Others will provide demonstration copies at a reduced cost. Whatever the arrangement, the purchaser should not have to pay full price until having had time to review the program.

Doing It Yourself

One of the comments heard most often at conferences involving computer applications is something similar to the following. "I have this great idea for a software package. All I have to do is find someone who will program it for me or learn to program it myself." While the author welcomes enthusiasm and the involvement of more persons in software development, a word of caution is appropriate. Developing a software package that has professional application is an arduous, time-consuming task. Chapter 12 contains a detailed discussion of what is involved. However, a few words are appropriate here.

The typical software package requires at least a year to prepare and field test. During this time the developer must be willing to return repeatedly to the program to make revisions. (And rewriting computer programs is about as much fun as rewriting term papers.)

Having someone else do the programming is difficult at best. And it requires more time and money than doing it yourself—more time in that there is not only the programmer's time to consider, but also the time it will take you to convey to the programmer what you want done. Moreover, the programmer must be one who will go back and make the changes—again a task for which few will have sustained enthusiasm.

There are now companies that are carrying software for communication disorders who have programmers on staff to work with people in the field.

This will lead to much faster and more efficient software development. Persons interested in doing it themselves, with the long-range goal of marketing the product, would do well to talk to these companies first. A list of software companies carrying products for persons in communicative disorders is found in Appendix B.

If users are interested in developing a program that is only going to be used in-house, or in controlled settings, and they have a professional programmer available, the product can be quite acceptable (Shipley, 1984). The value of in-house computer programs is that they can be individualized to meet specific needs and they can be modified as needs change. If the professional involved is in such a setting, developing special purpose software can be very rewarding and effective.

CONCLUDING STATEMENT

Professional development in any field today must include a component of training in the utilization of technology, and the field of communication disorders is no different in this regard. The serious professional should include in his professional development regimen an ongoing strategy for staying current on software development.

References

American Speech–Language–Hearing Association. (1984). Materials Section. *Asha*, **26**, 67–68.

Beyers, C., & Halcrow, A. (1984). What's behind the price of software? *Interface Age*, **9**, 59–63.

Boyle, B. (1984). Software performance evaluation. *Byte*, **9**, 175–188.

Chial, M. (1984). Evaluating microcomputer hardware. In A. Schwartz (Ed.), *Handbook of microcomputer applications in communication disorders*. San Diego: College-Hill Press.

Denning, P., & Brown, R. (1984). Operating systems. *Scientific American*, **251**, 94–129.

Fawcette, J. (1984). All you need to learn about programming. *Personal Computing*, **8**, 319–322.

Fitch, J. (1985). Software/hardware review policy. *Journal of Computer Users in Speech and Hearing*, **1**, 50.

Kay, A. (1984). Computer software. *Scientific American*, **251**, 52–59.

Lenat, D. (1984). Computer software for intelligent systems. *Scientific American*, **251**, 204–213.

Poole, L. (1981). *Apple II user's guide*. Berkeley, CA: Osborne/McGraw-Hill.

Poole, L. (1983). *Using your IBM personal computer*. Indianapolis: Howard W. Sams & Co.

Spector, A. (1984). Computer software for process control. *Scientific American*, **251**, 174–187.

4

The Human–Machine Interface

THE EVERYDAY INTERFACE

Occasionally a discussion of computers will lead someone to remark that "all that technology is frightening." A few years ago the author would have attributed that remark to be the belief that technology has the potential for being detrimental to mankind. Certainly there are bases for such a belief in the destructiveness of war weaponry and the fact that automobile accidents are a leading cause of death. However, the author now believes that the people making such remarks are generally not referring to the potential of technology to harm mankind, but in actuality are expressing their own fear of not knowing how the technology works. In other words, they are not afraid of the technology; what they fear is the possibility that they may not be able to control the technology.

This conclusion is based on the fact that these same people are generally as much involved in the day-to-day human–machine interface as everyone else. They awaken to an alarm clock, take a heated shower, fix breakfast using a stove, toaster, and coffee pot, drive to work in a car and use the typewriter, telephone, and other various "machines" in the course of the day. In the evening they watch television, attend a movie (driving a car to the theater, of course), dance to electronically amplified music, or even simply read a book at home (in the light of an electric lamp and in a room controlled by an automatic ventilation system). In other words, no one is exempt from living in the world of technology.

The fact is, technology has become so much a part of our lives that we take much of it for granted. Our food supply chain is completely dependent on technology. Animals are fed by machine-controlled feeders (now sometimes programmed by computers), transported to market in trucks, processed using a varied assortment of technology, canned by machines, or kept refrigerated until the consumer purchases them. They then go to the refrigerator of the consumer, later to be processed on his stove, oven, or microwave.

The airplane and automobile have become so much a part of our everyday lives that we also accept them as "natural" and "good." Most households have multiple television sets and radios and few people would decline the use of medical technology in the treatment of a serious disorder.

People who express a fear of technology often do not recognize that technology is a passive phenomenon. Technology by itself cannot be "good" or "bad," because it has no consciousness. It is simply a tool invented by man. The results of any technological development may be beneficial or detrimental to given individuals based on the manner in which they interact with it. To say that technology is bad because it reduces the amount of workers needed to produce a product can be countered by saying that it is good because it produces better products more efficiently and with less cost.

For years workers in many fields dreaded the advance of technology because they knew it would replace them in the workforce. Now many companies are recognizing this as a human problem, rather than a problem of technology, and are providing human solutions through retraining people for better jobs as technology begins to take over the old jobs. And intelligent workers today are mindful of the need for change and involve themselves in retraining throughout their careers.

The utilization of technology follows a pattern. Early in the development of any technological breakthrough, the procedures for using the technology and its price usually prevent widespread application. As the price falls, and the procedures for its use become simplified, the use broadens. Computers of the 1950s could accomplish most of the tasks to which we put the microcomputer today. However, the price and usability of the machine made its general application impractical. Applications have developed, and as the price and the procedures for using it have become within the reach of the professional in the field, the utilization of it as a clinical device has spread.

The parallel to everyday use of technology is also appropriate in considering the economics of technology. Most homes have the best technology that the owner can afford; i.e., the more expensive the house, the more current are the kitchen appliances, television sets, air conditioning and heating, etc. Computers have followed in the same pattern. However, since computers require more training to use than the kitchen stove or the television set, the price has had to become especially attractive to draw users. The agency purchasing computer equipment usually does so on the basis of usability and affordability. This is the way it should be.

THE PROFESSIONAL INTERFACE

Traditionally, computer technology has developed more quickly for business, science, and industrial applications than for applications involving human services. All of the above require processing of information and utilization of equipment that works in a consistent, logical, and definable manner. Perhaps it is for this reason that computers are last developed in the area of human interaction. Human interaction is extremely complex and often based on variables that are subject to only limited control.

Computers are programmed to complete specific functions. Interactions which require interpretation or interpolation of response, or which can deal with unusual and/or tangentially related response, are not easily programmable. (The author knows of no treatment program yet that responds appropriately when the patient says he has to use the bathroom.) The end result is that any interaction between a computer and a person requires that the person reduce response patterns to a limited number that the computer can recognize and act upon in a logical manner. This may change as the nature of computers develops more human-like capabilities, but for the present the role that the computer can play in human interaction is limited.

Attempts toward utilization of the computer with human behavior have had the most visibility in the field of education. The roles commonly ascribed to computer technology in that area are as follows:

1. Computer-assisted instruction
   a. Drill and practice
   b. Problem solving through simulation
2. Computer-based instruction (computer-managed instruction)
   a. Record management
   b. Electronic decision making
   c. Program planning

COMPUTER-ASSISTED INSTRUCTION

Drill and Practice

Computer-assisted instruction (CAI) through drill and practice exercises is the most common type of computer utilization. Teaching machines have been in evidence long before the computer. In the area of general language skills was the *PAL,* a program for language improvement that was originally designed for preschoolers but one that was adapted for adult aphasics (Katz, 1984). Drill and practice involves presenting a stimulus, soliciting a response, judging the response, and providing the patient with feedback concerning the correctness or appropriateness of the response. Drill and practice is usually considered appropriate and desirable when working with skills that need to be automatic, such as articulation, discrimination, or word recognition.

The computer is very well suited in the role of a drill and practice teaching machine. First of all, it can present stimuli in a variety of forms. It can present pictures or write words on the screen of the monitor, pictures can be programmed for action (movement), it can present spoken words through the speech synthesizer, and it can be programmed to control a variety of peripheral equipment such as videodisc systems and recorders. Second, it can be programmed to accept a variety of inputs, e.g., keyboard strokes, single switches, joysticks, word recognition systems, and others.

The limitation is in the range of stimuli and format for presentation and response. The stimuli must be somewhat structured and the response within a given mode. In addition, many of the special systems, such as speech recognition systems, require substantial capital outlay. While there are a number of drill and practice materials on the market (these will be discussed in Chapter 9), there will continue to be a need to develop more for years to come.

The primary advantage that the computer has when compared to its predecessor, the teaching machine, is that the computer can be programmed with artificial intelligence (AI) to respond with logic to client response patterns. For example, the computer can be programmed to present the client with progressively more difficult stimuli as the client masters the less difficult stimuli (Katz, 1984; Fitch, 1985). This will be discussed in more detail in Chapter 9.

Simulation

Computer-assisted instruction through simulation is based on presentation of real-life problems by the computer to which the user can respond.

The computer presents a situation to which the user reacts. The computer then changes the situation based on the response of the user. Simulation is the programming strategy used in video arcade games. For example, the video screen can display the picture of what the driver of a car or airplane actually sees, and then modify the picture based on how the user manipulates the controls. Many training facilities now employ computer-based instruction as a primary means of introducing skills before application in the field.

Many computer games employ the technique using words instead of pictures. The computer presents a situation and the user enters a response. Based on the response, the computer leads the user through a series of steps. Many computer games based on the concept of Dungeons and Dragons have used this strategy.

Simulation has several advantages in training programs. It allows the student to "practice" on the machine before administering the same procedure to a client. Probably the most common simulation in communication disorders is audiological testing. Several programs exist which simulate the testing paradigm. Students input the frequencies and intensities in the computer in the same manner in which they would test a client. The computer is programmed to respond in a variety of ways. It can simulate the responses of various types of hearing losses, normal hearing, malingering, etc.

Simulation permits the student to acquire experience without the problems associated with using human patients. Practice can be scheduled at the student's option, procedures can be repeated without inconvenience, and the computer can provide feedback on the accuracy of the testing technique. It is likely that simulation will come to play an important role in training programs.

COMPUTER-BASED INSTRUCTION

A Treatment Manager

Computer-based instruction (CBI) (O'Neil, 1981) is predicated on utilizing the computer as a manager of the educational process. Computer-based instruction (the term will be used interchangeably with computer-managed instruction in this book) includes using the computer to manage client files, assess behavior, develop programs of study, schedule activities, monitor performance, and generate reports (Baker, 1981). Under CBI systems, all information regarding the patient is stored on the computer. (However, the computer and client themselves never interact directly or indirectly in the assessment or treatment program as in computer-assisted instruction.) The computer is programmed to analyze response patterns and to recommend treatment prescriptions. At all levels the user (who should be a qualified professional) monitors the information and recommendations from the computer and makes the actual decisions on what will be done and how it will be done.

An Electronic Decision Maker

The computer, in this paradigm, is used to keep the records on an individual. It is programmed to make decisions based on specified, definable criteria. Then it completes the educational management process by generating course outlines, unit projects, lesson plans, and skills/objectives for the user to employ. The ultimate computer-based instruction system reduces the educational task to a series of discrete steps based on logical processing of learner characteristics and task analysis. It could be argued that the act of designing such a system would be more significant than the computerization of the model. As noted previously, probably the most important feature of using computers in behavioral change systems is found in the fact that to use the computers, tasks and behavioral characteristics must be analyzed in discrete, quantifiable terms. This requires users to analyze the treatment process in detail and through that analysis they will become more knowledgeable about the processes of treatment in their field.

Levels of Involvement

Just as the prospective homeowner decides how much technology he is going to include in the design of his home, clinicians have to decide how much of the clinical process they want to delegate to technology. The decisions, as indicated before, will be based on available funding, appropriateness of the available technology, and the knowledge that the user has concerning implementation of the technology. Initially, the amount of clinical utilization will be primarily dependent on funding and the availability of appropriate software. However, it will not be long before costs decrease and the amount of available software increases to the point that they will no longer be the primary considerations. In the end, the primary factor in determining the extent to which a clinic utilizes computers will be the skill and knowledge the professionals in that clinic have concerning computers. Furthermore, the credibility of agencies providing services for communication disorders will be based, in part, on the degree to which they have computerized operations. This will be strong motivation for clinics to provide their staffs with opportunities to develop computer skills.

At the present time, computer users can be grouped into four major classifications: administrative, clinical, application, development.

Administrative. Clinicians functioning in this role are able to operate general-purpose, commercially available software having to do with business applications (word processing, data management, spreadsheets). They use these programs to prepare diagnostic reports, keep client records, and manage the business operations of a clinical program. Most correspondence is generated through the word processor.

Clinical. Clinicians functioning in this role understand the basic operations of the computer and are aware of the strengths and limitations of the computer in clinical processes. They are aware of software that is available (both commercially and public domain) and can intelligently choose which software/hardware systems are appropriate for their clinical operations. Clinicians functioning at this level are able to critically review software to determine its worth to their operations.

Application. These persons have knowledge of the strength and limitations of the computer and are aware of the uses to which the computer can be applied in the field. They are current on existing software from several different areas and can coordinate the purchase and implementation of computer hardware and software. Although they may have only limited programming skills themselves, they are aware of how programs can be modified and can work with programmers in effecting modifications. They can plan and present workshops and in-service training for professionals in the field.

Development. Users in this role are knowledgeable about software or hardware that is available generally (not just to the field of communication disorders) and are able to apply that software or hardware to challenges within the field of communication disorders. They have command of one or more computer languages and have developed software that has found acceptance in the field. Persons functioning at this level have either had formal training in computers or have spent considerable time on their own developing computer expertise. Developers usually are well versed generally, but have special expertise in only one or two types of clinical applications in the field. For example, they may be proficient in applications in aphasia, but have limited expertise in other areas of computer applications.

Within each of the user roles—administrative, clinical, application, development—there are various skills levels. For practical purposes, users can be classified as beginner, intermediate, or advanced. Beginners are still at the level of having to focus attention primarily on the machine itself, i.e., how to load the program, which keys to press, and what to do to get a program to work.

Intermediate users can work the programs with ease and can use software as it is designed. In other words, instead of focusing on how the machine works, they focus on how the software works. They also have learned to troubleshoot minor problems.

Advanced users not only are able to use software in the way it was designed, but have found other uses as well. In addition, they integrate software to accomplish specific goals. Advanced users create systems which reflect their own perception of how the world should work. They do not have to focus on the hardware or software, but direct their attention to using the hardware and software to meet the needs of their own operations. They can troubleshoot all but major problems and can provide effective guidance and direction to other users.

At some point, clinicians will find themselves wanting to compare their own skills to that of others in the field generally. At this point such comparisons are difficult to specify because the field has no standards for assessing computer knowledge or skills for comparative purposes. At some point the field must recognize the need for computer knowledge or skills and incorporate it into the requirements for clinical competency.

TRAINING NEEDS

Steps Being Taken

Since it is evident that the field of communication disorders will make extensive utilization of the computer, it is imperative that those who shape the future of the profession recognize the need for inclusion of computer skills in training programs. This recognition is growing, as evidenced by the Committee Report of the American Speech–Language–Hearing Association's Ad Hoc Committee on Long-Range Planning (1983). One area studied for long-range planning was "major external factors likely to have a significant impact on the profession and its members in the next three to five years." At the top of the list was "the increasing role of computers and other technology." The address given by Minifie to the 1980 Directors of Graduate Training Programs Conference supported the need for increased opportunities for members, and prospective members, of the profession to learn to use computers.

The American Speech–Language–Hearing Association's leadership conferences on incorporating training in microcomputers in 1984 and 1985 were a major step toward encouraging universities to increase the amount of opportunities for computer training into their programs. While no statistics are available, the author is aware of many programs that have added, or modified, courses to include training in the use of computers.

The Challenge for Training Programs

There are two phases to the challenge for computer training. The first lies in updating university curricula in communication disorders to include greater amounts of computer training. It is suggested that all training programs will need to ensure that students have at least the administrative level of training to be competitive in the marketplace. Clinical positions in communication disorders require that considerable amounts of time be devoted to preparing reports, treatment plans, and general correspondence. The computer increases the efficiency of the individual in the field to the point that job applicants having computer skills will be given priority.

It is also suggested that to be considered for the top echelon of clinical positions, graduates will need to have the clinical level of expertise in addition to the administrative level. More and more clinical settings are purchasing computers for the purpose of direct, or indirect, provision of services. Obviously, a consideration in employing a person in that setting would be his skill in utilizing the available technology.

Persons who will be involved in designing and implementing computer services need to have a solid background in how computers work, and extensive exposure to clinical uses of software. At the present time, the person interested in developing skills in applications would need to draw from several resources, including computer science, education, business, and engineering.

The last level of training, that of developer of computer resources, also needs to be addressed by universities. Training programs need to recognize and make available resources and specially designed courses of study that allow the person who is interested in writing, developing, and field testing programs to achieve the skills needed to do so. At the present time few universities have the resources available to do this within departments of communication disorders. However, many settings have computer science departments that could provide the support, equipment, and expertise to guide the development of such a person. The field will have to extend itself to make available the necessary training opportunities to provide quality education for the advanced levels of computer skills. If the field does not do so, within a short time it will find itself with the problem that education faces. Osgood (1984) states that "Education suffers in the design loop: educators know what they want from software, but they can't write programs; programmers are not always versed in educational theory" (p.

161). If the field of communication disorders is to avoid becoming "slaves to someone else's technology" (Minifie, 1981), it must provide the opportunities for members of the field to achieve developer-level competence in computer skills.

Inherent in the above is the need for faculties to develop skills that can be translated into student training opportunities with computers. Already many faculties are seeing students entering college with more advanced computer skills than they themselves possess. Because of the special applications to the field, training cannot be delegated to the computer science department of the university. Very few will have courses, or personnel, who can make the student aware of the special human interface needs that members of the profession will require. Training programs must mandate levels of computer proficiency for faculties and while so doing, provide maximum opportunities for the development of those skills.

The Professional in the Field

The second phase of the problem of developing computer skills among members of the profession is more difficult. That problem is to reach the working professional who has completed training. The solution is to develop opportunities for those members of the profession to learn the computer skills that will they need to maintain the level of efficiency that will be demanded of them.

A professional in another field discussed the frustration at being a supervisor, with years of experience and recognition as a superior employee, who was suddenly faced with two entry-level workers who used word processing and completed their paperwork in half the time that it took the supervisor. While it did not detract from her own skills, her supervisor recognized that it took her longer to prepare reports than the new employees. After months of growing anxiety, and false attempts at self-study, she asked the younger members to help her learn how to use the computer. They were delighted to teach the supervisor, and within weeks she was able to prepare paperwork with the same efficiency.

The author had only one formal course in computer science. Most of the people with whom he has associated as programmers in the field have had no more training than that. And almost all would agree that one of the best ways to learn computer skills is to go where people with computer skills congregate. Over 50% of the computer skills that the author has developed can be attributed to the patient tutoring by individuals 15 years his junior. As more and more entry-level professionals in the field of communication disorders emerge from training institutions with computer skills, more and more expertise will be available through them to the person already in the field. If the person in the field will make the effort to tap that resource, the development of computer skills can be a natural and unpressured undertaking.

The author feels that there is a need for a national program with larger scope, aimed at providing training opportunities for the person already in the field. Regional centers with short-term intensive training may provide the answer. However, regardless of what opportunities are available, it is imperative that the professionals in the field be aware of, and make provisions for, developing computer skills that will permit them to move ahead with the rest of the profession.

INTERFACING TECHNOLOGY AND THE CLIENT

The profession must also develop strategies and skills for helping clinicians in the field teach clients to work with technology. It is recognized that clinicians must be the master of the technology and assign it only to the tasks for which it is especially well suited. Professionals must realize that the clinician is ultimately responsible for the welfare of the client. Technology does nothing to relieve them of that responsibility. Programs utilizing technology can only be effective if professionals use them intelligently.

The professional must also realize that clients may have the same apprehension toward technology that others have. One of the roles of clinicians is to help clients feel confident and comfortable working with technology, and to help them realize that behind it is a caring professional who can respond to their special, individual needs.

References

Ahl, D. (1983). The Turing Test: A historical perspective. *Creative Computing, 9,* 156–161.

Bonner, P. (1984). Computers in education: Promise and reality. *Personal Computing, 8,* 64–77.

Boyer, E. (1984). Education's new challenge. *Personal Computing, 8,* 81–85.

Cohen, C. (1984). Implementing microcomputer applications. In A. Schwartz (Ed.), *Handbook of microcomputer applications in communication disorders* (pp. 17–33). San Diego: College-Hill Press.

Committee Report, Ad Hoc Committee on Long-Range Planning. (1983). *Asha, 25,* 61–64. Pg 54

Emmett, A. (1983). American education: The dead end of the 80s. *Personal Computing, 7,* 97–105.

Emmett, A. (1983). Overcoming computer resistance. *Personal Computing, 7,* 80–93.

Fitch, J. (1985). *Computer managed articulation* treatment. Communication Skill Builders, Tucson, Arizona.

Katz, R. (1984). Using microcomputers in the diagnosis and treatment of chronic aphasic adults. *Seminars in Speech and Language, 5,* 11–12.

McGuire, D. (1983). Learning the hard way. *Personal Computing, 7*, 109–113.

Minifie, F. (1981). Graduate education during a technological revolution. *National Council of Graduate Programs in Speech and Language Pathology and Audiology Proceedings,* pp. 1–9. Rockville, MD.

Osgood, D. (1984). A computer on every desk. *Byte, 9*, 162–184.

Pournelle, J. (1983). The next five years in microcomputers. *Byte, 8*, 233–244.

Rosenwald, P. (1985). Computing's agony and ecstasy. *Personal Computing, 9*, 227–228.

Rothfeder, J. (1983). Striking back at technological terror. *Personal Computing, 7*, 62–66.

Rubin, C. (1983). Some people should be afraid of computers. *Personal Computing, 7*, 55–57, 163.

Shearer, W. (1984). Academic and instruction applications for microcomputers. In A. Schwartz (Ed.), *Handbook of microcomputer applications in communication disorders* (pp. 193–218). San Diego; College-Hill Press.

Toong, H., & Gupta, A. (1982). Personal computers. *Scientific American, 247*, 86–107.

5

Word Processing

A PROFESSIONAL NECESSITY

The importance of being able to handle paperwork efficiently is such that all professionals who are required to prepare reports, letters, grant applications, and other word-related efforts should consider training on word processing a necessity. They should at least be required to provide their secretaries with word processors. However, for professionals with competent typing skills, the word processor itself has become a secretary of sorts.

The phrase word processor can be used in two different contexts: one as hardware and one as software. Word processing is the electronic manipulation of words to construct documents. *Document* refers to any printed material: letters, contracts, reports, etc. It requires special software, which is sometimes referred to as a "word processor" or "word processing package." Word processing software is available for all types of computers, so there is no special hardware required. However, sometimes the computers that are dedicated to the task of word processing are called "word processors." They may have special keys and other functions that make them easier to use with word processing software. In this book, *word processor* will refer to the software.

ADVANTAGES OF WORD PROCESSING

People with the nicest words to say about word processors are those who use them daily. Those who use them only sporadically may have reserved judgment. The word processor is a computer program that allows the user to manipulate words without having to know a computer language. The word processing software itself, however, has commands to learn. In the top of the line, do-it-all word processing software, there are well over 100 commands. Even the low end word processing software packages have over 50 commands.

People who have heard about the power of word processors are often disappointed in the early stages of use because they spend more time looking up commands than inputting information. And a wrong command can wipe out hours of typing. It takes a while before the moaning and wailing about lost and/or damaged documents gives way to sighs of relief. But once the user becomes skilled in operating the word processor, the savings in time and effort are manifest and the conversion to digital writing is complete. It is somewhat like learning to ride a bike: the first few falls make the prospective user wonder if it is worth it, but once mastered it is a source of pride and enjoyment.

Administrative Benefits

Typical comments made in reference to using word processors comes from administrative personnel who do not know how to type: "Since I can't type, what good is the word processor?" And "Since I have a good secretary, why do I need a word processor?" It is agreed that not being able to type limits one's potential for using the computer in any capacity. And if an individual has a secretary who does this type of work, then having a word processor does not make his job easier—only the secretary's job.

Individuals who have secretaries who are organized and efficient are indeed fortunate. While the word processor will not replace secretaries, it will make their work easier and give them the capability of completing work faster and more efficiently. It should be recognized that a word processor reduces the time that it takes to prepare documents by over 50%, and document storage and retrieval are faster. And the speed, accuracy, and appearance of clerical work in an office reflects on the supervisor.

Administrators who claim they are "decision makers" and that they have others to "do the work" are rapidly losing ground due to the fact that information for decision making now is contained in databases. The ability to make decisions today is, to a degree, predicated on an individual's ability to access databases and obtain information. The individual who is dependent on someone else for information will be at a disadvantage. (Databases will be discussed in the next chapter.)

Furthermore, the integration of information from databases with the report preparation capabilities of word processing leads to reports that are outstanding in quality. More young professionals than ever are using microcomputers for the database and word processing capabilities. In the near future, virtually all young persons entering any profession will use these features of the computer. The professional in the field will need to develop word processing skills to remain competitive in the administrative domain.

Word processing is increasingly being used in conjunction with electronic communication systems. Electronic communication systems, or *networking*, is a system through which memorandums and office notes can be generated on networked computers. The ability to communicate with the rest of an agency's staff may be dependent on the individual's ability to use word processing in conjunction with the networking capability of microcomputers.

One small, but very important advantage of word processing is that it allows for very efficient editing. The word processor does not greatly decrease the amount of time that it takes to prepare the first copy of an original document. It still must be typed in (although word processors that accept spoken input are available for limited vocabulary). However, once the original document is stored, it can be called up time and time again for modification and use. Because of the editing capability, all correspondence coming from the word processor can be revised until letter perfect, thereby reducing the flow of correction fluid to nothing. The professional appearance of documents composed on a word processor enhances the professional image of an office.

Moreover, since editing is easy, there is a tendency to do more of it. There is sometimes a second thought given to handing a secretary a letter which has been prepared just as requested, but in which a wording change is desired that will alter a line and require retyping the whole document. There is no such hesitancy when a word processor is involved because of the ease with which the change can be made.

Most professionals in the field of communication disorders have to rely on their own clerical skills to a great extent. For them the word processor will represent a significant tool for increasing efficiency.

HOW THEY WORK

There are several different formats for word processors and several different types of functions. This chapter will deal with word processors in the generic sense. Whenever a function described is not standard in word processing programs, it will be noted. It must be recognized that word processing is still a developing field and by the time this manuscript is published, there will undoubtedly be many changes.

Getting It Started

A few word processors are now stored on a ROM (read-only memory) chip in the computer, thus allowing the program to be loaded in when the computer is turned on. However, most word processing software is stored on diskettes. Some word processing packages require two disk drives and some only one. Those that require two disk drives utilize one drive to move information to the computer from the program diskette and the other to store documents. The second diskette is usually referred to as the *data diskette* to differentiate it from the *program diskette*. Those with one drive load the program from the program diskette. The program diskette is then removed from the drive and a data diskette inserted when the user wants to store a document.

Some word processing software requires the user to configure the system (tell how many disk drives, type of printer, etc.) initially. This configuration can then be changed when different equipment is used.

Once configured, the user can then begin to prepare the document by typing in content (sometimes referred to as *text*). Time is saved in text entry (in comparison to the typewriter) primarily because of two features. The first time-saving feature is that the typist does not have to keep track of line length and hit a return key at the end of the line. Text entry is continuous and line length is calculated by the computer. Many word processing programs have the capability of formatting the document on the screen the same way that it will come out on the printer. Other programs, however, will show only continuous text which will be divided into lines of appropriate length when output to a printer.

A second time-saving feature of word processing is the use of stored material. This is particularly significant in documents that have redundant wording. For example, a diagnostic report usually has a great deal of redundant material. Words, phrases, sentences, and paragraphs such as the following are commonly found in diagnostic reports: "articulation," "hearing loss," "within normal limits," "The patient was seen at the Speech and Hearing Clinic on referral from," and "The clinician met with the parent and discussed the policies and procedures of the Speech and Hearing Clinic, including fees, procedures for notifying the clinic an absence is anticipated and clinic observation policies. The release of information form was explained to the parent who signed it." Any of these could be inserted with as few as four keystrokes. That represents a savings of 66% in keystrokes for the word *articulation* and a savings of 98.5% for the paragraph. Obviously, the more redundant the information, the more efficient the word processor is in preparing documents.

In addition, tabs can be set for material and automatic indenting of paragraphs can be employed. When all these features are used together, there is substantial savings on entering original documents. The real time savings, however, come in the editing capability.

Editing

Once a document is written, it is easy to make changes. Documents are stored on diskettes and can be entered into the computer in seconds. Letters, words, sentences, paragraphs, etc. can be inserted without disturbing or retyping any of the text.

Editing is usually accomplished by moving the cursor (flashing square or underline) to the point at which the change is to be made. In the edit mode, this can be accomplished without disturbing the surrounding text. When at the editing point, material can be erased, changed, or inserted with equal ease. When editing is complete, the document can be saved on the data diskette in the new form. It can be saved as a replacement for the document changed, or saved as a new document, allowing the old one to be stored in its original form.

One feature of editing that can save tremendous amounts of time is the search/replace function. A command is given to put the word processor in search/replace mode. Then the material that is to be changed and the change that is to be made are entered. The computer searches the manuscript for each occurrence of the material to be replaced and signals it on the screen. The user has the option of either replacing the material in the document or going to the next occurrence. This allows for some occurrences to be changed while others are retained.

Many programs have a global change function. Using it, the user can tell the computer to replace all occurrences of one portion of the text with another. An example would be the rewriting of a letter in which you wanted to change the name from Jones to Smith. No matter how many times Jones is mentioned in the text, it would be changed to Smith instantaneously.

The ease with which editing can be accomplished encourages the user to edit more thoroughly than when using a typewriter. And, of course, it leads to a more rapidly produced document.

Printing the Document

Printing a document on a printer requires a very short time and the product reflects a professional effort. This in turn enhances a professional image. The printing routines available in word processing permit a wide range of formatting that encourages experimentation. For example, a document can be printed first in pica, then elite print, to determine which has the best appearance for that particular material. It can be done in boldface print and print expanded to various degrees. Some routines include several different *fonts,* or styles of print. It takes only a short time (and a few sheets of paper), and the result can be a document that is greatly improved by its printing format. To make the changes from one to another requires only a few keystrokes to give instructions to the printer.

Line length, paragraph indentation, centering material, line spacing, and page numbering are other parameters which can be changed in the printout without retyping any of the text. Dot matrix printers may also have the capability of graphics, that is, the ability to print dots in patterns to form recognizable images. Pictures, graphs, and charts can be incorporated into the output of some word processors. However, graphics usually require the use of separate software.

SYSTEM INTERACTION FUNCTIONS

The more powerful word processing packages are systems that include the interaction of two or more programs. Some of the functions that can be generated can save huge amounts of time and effort.

Form Letters

One of the most powerful is that of the personalized form letter. It is estimated that today over 90% of the mail is computer generated. Form letters are generated in the following manner. First, the basic letter is written, with codes in those places which will be changed in each letter: name, address, salutation, etc. Then a file is created which contains only the names, addresses, salutations, etc., with a code identifying each element. A master program then controls the printout by including coded material where indicated and filling in the text as written. A great many form letters can be printed in a relatively short time using the word processor.

Mail Merge

An extention of this function is the mail merge function. Mail merge software work in the following manner. A master list of all the names and addresses is stored in the mail merge program. Each file contains as much information as desired on the individual. The information is stored in *fields* with codes, or names, such as first name, last name, street, city, zip code, occupation, profession, age, sense of humor. The information can be put into the field in any form desired.

Once the master list is built, it can be printed on labels in its entirely or the program can print labels for only selected individuals. For example, it can be specified to print only the addresses of those who are over 30 years of age and have the word "yes" written in the "married" field. This saves hours of sorting records and typing labels.

For more organized administrative applications, the lists can be printed out in alphabetical order, according to name (or any other field). Those who occasionally have the need to utilize bulk mailing will like the feature which allows the user to print out labels in numerical sequence according to zip code.

Spell Checkers

Professionals who prepare material for publication may want to use word processors that have spelling checking capability. The spelling checking programs have dictionaries of words which are compared to the words in the text. If the spelling program does not find a word in the dictionary to match the spelling of a word in the text, this is indicated to the user. The user can add words to the dictionary which the program will thereafter include when checking for spelling. This is usually necessary for individuals whose writing includes a great deal of professional vocabulary. Programs which check grammar and syntax are beginning to appear in the marketplace, but as yet are not widespread.

Most of the interactive programs require extra software and can be used only in conjunction with certain word processing packages. The greater the number of users to which the system can be applied, the more savings are accrued to the user.

ORGANIZING FILES

As a daily word processor user, and as an individual whose organizational skills are highly suspect, the author finds one of the most useful aspects of word processing to be the organization that it brings to the desk top. First of all, the amount of paper that is used to produce a manuscript is drastically reduced using the word processor. Typically the author does two to three rewrites of a manuscript before putting it on paper. The first draft on paper is then rewritten and the word processor used to edit the rewrite. Often other people read the manuscript and make recommendations for changes as well. This sequence continues until an acceptable product is obtained. While as many as 10 draft versions of the manuscript are generated, only two or three are actually printed on paper before getting to the final product. The cutting, pasting, and stapling of modifications are eliminated, making writing a much more tolerable and more organized task.

Another organizing feature of the word processor is the manner in which files are maintained. Using the traditional paper files, a need to retrieve a previously generated document meant a trip to the file cabinet and an exercise in patience to try to track it down. Computer files are much easier. The author stores his documents on diskettes labeled for the general subject area, i.e., course material, presentations, CUSH correspondence, etc. The individual documents are coded by short names indicative of content. For example, letters to individuals are coded by the name of the individual, and agencies by their names. A second letter to an agency will have a "2" following the name, a third letter a "3," and so on.

After the disk is inserted, two keystrokes project the names of the documents on the screen. A listing for a complete diskette (which may contain 20–40 documents) can be viewed in seconds. Once the correct one is identified, it can be input to the computer from the diskette in seconds.

Misfiling can be a problem; the author has a tendency to store things on the most accessible data diskette. While this sometimes means searching several diskettes to find the right document, it is far easier than searching through several files jammed with paper.

With its built-in organizational advantages, and the ease of editing, the word processor is a forgiving tool; that is, it is one that allows the user to make mistakes without suffering too greatly. To those of us who are prone to making mistakes, it is truly a thing to cherish.

CLINICAL APPLICATIONS

Some Considerations

Most clinicians would agree that one of the least popular tasks in the profession is the preparation of reports. Later in this section there is an example of how a word processor can be used to reduce the amount of effort that goes into creating a diagnostic report. Before looking at the sample, however, there needs to be a discussion of the factors that go into a report.

The computer will not directly improve the quality of a report (other than looks). The computer should be viewed as only a means of getting the information on paper quickly and in an organized fashion. If the evaluation process itself is not organized, the report will reflect that lack of organization.

Report formats vary tremendously. Some take the form of abbreviated checklists while others use elaborate narrative forms. The computer should not dictate the format of the report. Members of an agency seeking to use computers in the report process should consider first what they want the report to be. Then they should determine how the computer can help. Generally the savings gained by the word processor will be in proportion to the length and complexity of the report format.

An Example

Figure 7 is an example for discussion purposes. It is a report that follows basically a narrative form. The words that are bracketed indicate character strings that are input to the text with one or two key strokes using a glossary function (which will be discussed shortly).

If the entire report had been typed, almost 2000 keystrokes would have been required. Using the word processor with the glossary function, the number of keystrokes was reduced to less than half. This means a savings of over 50% in the mechanical text entry process. Additional savings are gained when correcting errors. Correcting a typographical error with the word processor requires only a few keystrokes, but correction of a typed version requires considerably more time and effort, and a correction on the typewriter *looks* like a correction. With the computer, the user can keep making changes until the document looks as desired, and then print it.

Setting It Up

The report above takes advantage of the ability of the computer to store strings of characters (words, phrases, sentences, and even paragraphs) and quickly retrieve them and incorporate them into the text. This is sometimes called the *glossary* function. It works in this way. First, the user goes over reports that have been previously written to determine redundant elements. Redundant parts (words, phrases, sentences, paragraphs) are then written in a separate file called a glossary. Each entry is coded with a letter. When the user wishes to use a word from the glossary, the glossary option is called (one or two keystrokes) and the specific item from the glossary is entered into the text with one or two more keystrokes. The more redundancy to the reports, the more efficient the glossary function.

(SPEECH AND HEARING CLINIC
UNIVERSITY OF SOUTH ALABAMA
MOBILE, ALABAMA 36688)

(NAME:) Williamson, Tony   (SEX:) M   (DOB:)   3/30/82
(ADDRESS:) 714 West Maple Street
           Anytown, USA 00000
(PARENTS:) M&M. William Williamson   (PHONE:) 000-0000
(CLASSIFICATION:) Articulation   (DOE:) 5/5/88
(REFERRED BY:)   Dr. Sam Smith
(FILE NUMBER:)   00-0000

(BACKGROUND:)

     (This child was seen at the University Speech and Hearing
Clinic on) May 5, 1988. Tony (was referred by) Dr. Sam Smith,
Pediatrician, (for an evaluation of) communication skills.

(CASE HISTORY:)

   Tony's mother reported delayed developmental milestones,
e.g., taking first steps at 16 months and saying first words at
18 months. It was reported that he has had a history of ear
infections. No other significant health problems were noted.
According to his mother, Tony's eating and sleeping habits are
well regulated. Tony has two older sisters with whom it is
reported he interacts well. He plays with neighborhood
children daily. No problems other than that the other children
have some difficulty understanding him were reported.

(TESTS ADMINISTERED AND RESULTS:)

     (Articulation:) Tony's (articulation) was marked by
(distortion)s, (substitution)s and some (omission)s. ((See the
attached Articulation Test for specific errors.)) (The
intelligibility of his speech is judged to be) 75%. Tony (was
easily understood when the topic of the conversation was
known.) Tony was (stimulable) on all (sound)s. (It appears the
misarticulations are functional in nature so the prognosis for
remediation is good.)

(OBSERVATIONS:)

     Tony (was cooperative during the evalution. He followed
directions well and maintained attention to the task.) On one
occasion he was distracted when there was noise in the hallway
outside the clinic room. It appears that Tony (will respond
well in a treatment program.)

(RECOMMENDATIONS:)

     1. (A complete audiological evaluation is recommended.)

     2. (It is recommended that the child be enrolled·in a
treatment program) as soon as possible.

(Jane E. Doe, M.S.
Speech Pathologist-CCC)

Figure 7. A report constructed on word processor.

```
                     SPEECH AND HEARING CLINIC
                     UNIVERSITY OF SOUTH ALABAMA
                     MOBILE, ALABAMA   36688


NAME:                                        SEX:      DOB:

ADDRESS:


PARENTS:                                     PHONE:

CLASSIFICATION:                              DOE:

REFERRED BY:

FILE NUMBER:


BACKGROUND:


TESTS ADMINISTERED AND RESULTS:


OBSERVATIONS:


RECOMMENDATIONS:



Jane E. Doe, M.S.
Speech Pathologist-CCC
```

Figure 8.   An example of a report format.

Some word processing packages include report formats. "Fields" of information, such as identifying information, may be stored in a report format. Figure 8 is an example of a report format. Report preparation begins by loading the format and completing the information. The program starts with the cursor in the correct position for the first character in the field "NAME." When the name has been entered, the user strikes the RETURN key and the cursor jumps to the correct position in the next field, in this case "SEX." The body of the report is such that any desired information can be entered. The user can type in as much individualized text as desired and use the glossary function only when appropriate.

Figure 9 is a listing of the glossary for the example letter in Fig. 7. Using

```
aarticulation
AArticulation
bsubstitution
cA conference was held to discuss the results of the
evaluation.
CThe child was accompanied to the Clinic by
ddistortion
fNo treatment is recommended at this time.
gIt is recommended that the child be enrolled in a
treatment program
hA complete audiological evaluation is recommended.
iA psychological evaluation is recommended.
IThe intelligibility of his speech was judged to be
mstimulable
MIt appears the misarticulations are functional in nature
so the prognosis for remediation is good.
nwas cooperative during the evaluation.  He followed
directions well and maintained attention to the task.
rWill respond well in a treatment program.
ssound
S(See the attached Articulation Test for specific
errors.)
tThis child was seen at the University Speech and Hearing
Clinic on
uwas referred by
Uwas easily understood when the topic of the conversation
was known.
vfor an evaluation of
```

Figure 9.   The glossary of the letter in Fig. 7.

the author's word processor, a sentence such as "Susan was easily understood when the topic of the conversation was known" would be actually typed on the computer as "Susan (control-G, U)." Without the glossary function 72 keystrokes would be required. With the glossary function the number is reduced to 7 keystrokes.

It is important to note that using the word processor in no way detracts from the individuality of the report. Users can include as much individuality as they wish.

Doing It Your Way

Report preparation is probably the most visible and time-saving use of word processing. The user should take time to learn the capabilities of the word processor and then study the report format that is desired. With some careful planning, the time required for report preparation can be reduced significantly.

References

Emmett, A. (1984). Picking the perfect word processor. *Personal Computing*, **8**, 112–192.
Heintz, C. (1984). Sifting through the word processing maze. *Interface Age*, **9**, 46–54, 113–123.
Heintz, C. (1984). To integrate or not to integrate. *Interface Age*, **9**, 76–81, 130–138.
Hood, S., & Miller, L. (1984). Administrative applications for microcomputers. In A. Schwartz (Ed.), *Handbook of microcomputer applications in communication disorders* (pp. 219–245). San Diego: College-Hill Press.
Naiman, A. (1984). Evaluating word-processing programs. *Byte*, **9**, 243–246.
Pagnoni, M. (1984). Bank Street Writer. *Byte*, **9**, 282–284.
Special Section. (1984). Everything you ever wanted to know about word processing. *Computers and Programs*, **1**, 92–121.
Zarley, C. (1983). Making mailing lists more personal. *Personal Computing*, **7**, 85–93.

6

Data Processing

IMPORTANCE OF ACCOUNTABILITY

The first widespread use of the computer was in business. The reason, of course, was that the computer is very well disposed toward the processing of numbers. The manipulation of numbers, when used in reference to computers, is called *data processing*.

Originally the computer was used to do the things that had been done by hand before the computer. In the business world this was keeping accounting books and inventory lists. The focus of such tasks is accountability, or maintaining a record of what has been done. Money that has been received or spent must be accounted for in order for the businessman to know where he stands financially. Inventories must be maintained in order for him to know what to buy. Without this information a businessman cannot stay in business.

For many years, persons in the field of communication disorders functioned without the benefit of such knowledge. They were employed in school and community clinics that were funded by outside sources. By and large those sources did not question the operation of the service and accountability was not required. Recently, however, that has begun to change. Funding sources are being stretched and many places now face the task of reducing services. In order to make an intelligent decision about cuts, the funding organization must have information on the operation. They must know who is accomplishing what with whom.

Accountability is a word that has steadily crept into the everyday vernacular of the profession. It is probably here to stay. Those who are to survive will have to be able to provide evidence that what they do justifies the continued existence of their positions.

Accountability for Leadership

There is another facet to accountability. Many persons in the field assume roles that require administrative skills. Clinic managers, department heads, and supervisors are in decision-making positions that require a business-oriented approach. In addition to the above roles, private practice is a growing area of the profession and one that requires more than passing expertise in accountability. Those who are to achieve leadership positions in the profession will have to develop and maintain accountability strategies.

TYPES OF DATA PROCESSING

At the present time, data processing can be broken into two major categories: electronic spreadsheets and electronic file management systems (databases). Both the concepts of data processing have been thoroughly tested and have histories dating back to the beginning of business per se. The computer does not so much change the system as make the system more efficient to use through the electronic manipulation of information.

SPREADSHEETS

Spreadsheets traditionally are long sheets of paper on which are placed rows and columns of data. Business reports and inventory lists require such compilation of data in relatively specific forms. Spreadsheets have the built-in advantage of a checking system. By adding the sums of the rows and comparing that to the sums of the columns, the user can ensure that the figures were added correctly. While this was an important feature for spreadsheets before computers, the accuracy of the computer eliminates the need to check arithmetic operations.

An Example

Figure 10 is a spreadsheet composed for a fictitious speech and hearing clinic. It gives a breakdown of the work load and amount of money gen-

MONTHLY REPORT

PLEASANT HILL SPEECH & HEARING CLINIC

DIAG	CLIN 1			CLIN 2			CLIN 3			TOTAL		
	NR	HRS	AMT$	NR	HRS	AMT$	NR	HRS	AMT$	NR	HRS	AMT$
SP/LN	2	4	80	6	12	240	5	8	180	13	24	500
OTHER	0	0	0	0	0	0	7	11	350	7	11	350
TRTMNT												
ARTIC	8	32	640	16	48	960	4	16	320	28	96	1920
LANG	12	84	1680	2	16	320	0	0	0	14	100	2000
FLNCY	4	10	200	0	0	0	2	8	160	6	18	360
VOICE	0	0	0	8	48	960	0	0	0	8	48	960
REHAB	0	0	0	0	0	0	7	11	220	7	11	220
TOTAL	26	130	2600	32	124	2480	25	54	1230	83	308	6310

Figure 10. An example of a spreadsheet for a clinic.

erated for each of the three clinicians employed by the clinic. An analysis of the spreadsheet gives the reader a relatively complete idea of how the clinicians spent their time that month. It can be noted that clinician 1 and clinician 2 generated twice the amount of revenue generated by clinician 3. Such a breakdown can permit the reader to compare clinicians and services with regard to the amount of revenue generated. While there are obviously other factors to be considered, this type of data can be of value in making intelligent decisions on personnel utilization.

As indicated before, the concept of the spreadsheet is not new; it has been used in business operations for many years. The advantage of electronic spreadsheets is the reduced amount of preparation time. Obviously the user could have a printed blank report form in which the figures for the month could be entered manually. Totals could be determined by entering the figures into a calculator. This, however, is time consuming. The computer, on the other hand, calculates the totals almost instantaneously and with virtually complete accuracy. The gains in time savings and accuracy of data are enormous, while the ease with which this type of report can be generated increases the likelihood that it will be done. The increased accountability gives the user more information on which to base decisions. The spreadsheet is the ideal way to indicate to the board of directors of a clinic the need for increased manpower (given that the figures warrant increased manpower).

Forecasting the Future

As stated before, accountability is a process of keeping track of what has happened in order to understand how an operation works. It provides a perspective in retrospect. That perspective is important for understanding the operation and forms the basis for making decisions concerning the future.

Knowledge of what has occurred is obviously important when making a decision concerning the future. However, by itself, it does not indicate what will necessarily happen in the future. Intelligent decisions about the future of an operation depend on the ability of the person making the decision to conceptualize the future. Conceptualizing the future depends on the person's ability to predict what will happen.

In business, the computer has become an important tool in predicting what will happen in the future. While the computer cannot make predictions per se, it can be used to indicate how the numbers will change given certain conditions. This allows the user to create ''what if'' scenarios that will indicate how the numbers will change given changes in parameters of the operation.

An Example

The following example shows how the computer can be used to make ''what if'' projections. A prospective budget for equipment has been prepared. To reconcile the actual budgeted amount ($116,000) with the proposed budget ($128,200), the user employs the ''what if'' strategy. Figure 11A shows the first budget. In it the user proposed the budget for the next year with a breakdown for each line item. The total of the proposed budget, the actual amount budgeted, and the difference are presented. Then changes are made by putting new figures in for the items. As the new amount for each line item is inserted, the totals and difference are recalculated. Figure 11B indicates how the screen would look after the budget is reconciled.

In effect the user is asking ''what will the total be if each of the elements cost. . . .'' Obviously this type of calculating when developing a budget must be done regardless of whether one has a computer or not. The computer simply makes the task easier, faster, and more accurate. It reduces the time it takes the user to add the figures on a calculator. Anyone who has had to complete budgets can appreciate this feature.

For more elaborate problems, the computer is even more more important. Suppose an agency is told that due to budget deficits, the existing budget is being prorated. (This problem has an all-too-familiar ring to many of us.) If the amount of proration is 5%, then each line item must be

A		B	
YEARLY BUDGET		YEARLY BUDGET	
SALARIES	72000	SALARIES	72000
FRINGE BENEFITS	24000	FRINGE BENEFITS	24000
FACILITY MAINT.	12000	FACILITY MAINT.	6600
UTILITIES	4000	UTILITIES	3600
TELEPHONE	3000	TELEPHONE	1200
INSURANCE	1200	INSURANCE	1200
EQUIPMENT	2400	EQUIPMENT	1800
SUPPLIES/OFFICE	3600	SUPPLIES/OFFICE	2400
SUPPLIES/PROF.	6000	SUPPLIES/PROF.	3200
TOTAL	128200	TOTAL	116000
BUDGETED	116000	BUDGETED	116000
DIFFERENCE	-12200	DIFFERENCE	0

Figure 11. An example of (A) a budget worksheet and (B) the completed budget proposal after reconciliation.

recalculated by that percentage. With the information on the present budget in a computerized spreadsheet, this can be done with one instruction and the task completed in less than a minute—regardless of how many line items are being changed. In a year in which 10% increases are granted (to assume a positive scenario), new budgets can be calculated from old ones with the same efficiency.

While giving a workshop at another institution, the author showed the chairman of the communication disorders department how to use a spreadsheet. The next week the chairman called to thank me. He indicated that in the first use of the spreadsheet, which had been to calculate the personnel costs (state and federal income tax, social security, etc.) for the next year, he was able to do in 2 hours what had previously taken about 2 days. Similar savings are reported by others.

DATABASE MANAGERS

Database managers are software programs which can be used to manage nonnumerical data in much the same way that spreadsheets manage numerical data. Database managers maintain file systems which permit the rapid and efficient retrieval of information.

Database software differs considerably in organization from the spreadsheet, which has a relatively standard format. There are different types of database systems for accomplishing different types of tasks. The most common type of database software is that of file management. In file management systems, the information is input to the database in much the same way that information would be put into any organized file. The database is composed of records (which are analogous to clinic folders on clients) on which all information on one individual, agency, or item is put into one storage area. The record is broken into "fields" (name, age, sex, etc.). The number and labels of the fields are determined by the user.

The records can then be retrieved from the database through sort routines. Sort routines are computer functions that permit information to be retrieved based on certain characteristics. In a clinic operation, it would be a simple matter to retrieve through a database all records of individuals over 60 years old who were referred for alaryngeal speech training. Obviously the same type of sorting could be done by hand by clerical staff, but as with most operations, the computer is superior in terms of being faster and more accurate. An example of a file management database will be demonstrated later in the chapter.

There are other database systems in addition to file management databases. Some of the more common ones are (1) relational databases; (2) hierarchical databases; (3) network databases; (4) free-format databases. Whereas the file management databases are limited to sort and retrieve routines, relational databases can combine records which have common fields. Hierarchical databases are like relational ones, but the data are not broken into fields. All data in one record are linked simply by the fact that it is included in that record. Rather than sort and retrieve, the links are fixed at the time that the file is initiated.

Network databases work in the same manner as hierarchical ones, but permit more than one link between records—whereas all data in one record has a link only to that record in hierarchical databases, network databases permit many links to many records. Free-format databases permit information to be input in any amount and any form. Each record is tagged with keywords which later allow for the retrieval of that information. A book with an index is an example of a free format database. The reader is referred to an excellent article in *Byte* magazine (Krajewski, 1984) for a more complete description of types of databases.

An Example

Figures 12 through 15 are examples of how a database software system may be used in a clinical operation. The actual database is a listing of hearing aid fittings for the year of 1985. The average practitioner would have considerably more entries, but the example contains enough to demonstrate what can be done.

This database was completely assembled using a user-friendly software package. Initially, the database program asks for the categories (fields) to be included in a record. Figure 12 is how the screen looks after the fields were chosen. Many more categories (in this database over 250) could have been added; those in Fig. 12 are examples only. The computer accepts entries for each field until all fields have been filled. Then it moves to a blank form again so that another record can be inserted. Making a new record is just a matter of putting in new information.

When all the records have been completed, a readout can be requested. Figure 13 demonstrates how the database program rearranges the information from each record and puts it all into one document. Whether the user has 10, as in this example, or several hundred, the computer will print the information as fast as the printer can print.

The completed database then can be sorted for specified characteristics. For example, a sort to identify all persons who were fitted with BTE100 aids and all who were fitted with ITE100 aids could be requested. The information would be printed as in Fig. 14. The database demonstrated here also permits sorting according to date. Suppose the user would like a listing of all hearing aid fittings performed before July 1, 1985. The result of such a sort is seen in Fig. 15. Sorts can also be performed using multiple variables. For example, the user could request a list of persons who were seen between May and September, who had a moderate hearing loss, and who were not fitted with a hearing aid.

It was indicated earlier that one definition of a computer is "something on which things are done that would not be done without a computer." In this case, the information that is available is the same type of information

```
Name:
Address:
City:
State:
Zip:
Telephone:
Loss-Type:
Loss-Degree:
Hearing Aid:
Date Fitted:
```

Figure 12. An example of format for a hearing aid evaluation database.

File: H. Aid Database
Report: H. Aid Fittings

Name	Address	City	State	Zip	Telephone	Loss-Type	Loss-Degree	Hrng Aid	Date Fitted
Atkins, Maudie	100 New Lane	Centerville	AL	36666	111-1111	S/N	Moderate	BTE100	Jan 1 85
Barlow, Homer	Newton Road	Newburgh	AL	36600	222-2222	S/N	Severe	BA100	Feb 2 85
Cuthbert, Calvin	200 North Road	Fishtown	AL	33660	333-3333	Mixed	Moderate	BTE100	Mar 3 85
Dalton, Leroy	303 Timber Lane	Hopetown	AL	36601	444-4444	Conductive	Mild	No	
Horton, Maxine	400 Happy Acres	Water Port	AL	36030	555-5555	Mixed	Moderate	ITE100	May 5 85
Lawrence, Warren	505 Grand Blvd.	View City	AL	36699	666-6666	Conductive	Moderate	BTE100	Jun 6 85
Quinton, Minnie	6000 Sap Run	Oak Haven	AL	36688	777-7777	S/N	Moderate	BTE100	Jul 7 85
Theodore, Arnie	4004 Maple St.	Forrestdale	AL	36677	888-8888	Mixed	Moderate	No	
Wellington, Biff	1 Porter House	Steak Island	AL	36661	999-9999	S/N	Moderate	ITE100	Sep 9 85
Xenia, Phoebe	414 Scary Lane	Spook City	AL	36679	000-0000	Mixed	Moderate	ITE100	Oct 10 85

Figure 13. Hearing aid evaluation database with information entered.

File: H. Aid Database
Report: H. Aid Fittings
Selection: Hrng Aid equals BTE100
or   Hrng Aid equals ITE100

Name	Address	City	State	Zip	Telephone	Loss-Type	Loss-Degree	Hrng Aid	Date Fitted
Atkins, Maudie	100 New Lane	Centerville	AL	36666	111-1111	S/N	Moderate	BTE100	Jan 1 85
Cuthbert, Calvin	200 North Road	Fishtown	AL	33660	333-3333	Mixed	Moderate	BTE100	Mar 3 85
Horton, Maxine	400 Happy Acres	Water Port	AL	36030	555-5555	Mixed	Moderate	ITE100	May 5 85
Lawrence, Warren	505 Grand Blvd.	View City	AL	36699	666-6666	Conductive	Moderate	BTE100	Jun 6 85
Quinton, Minnie	6000 Sap Run	Oak Haven	AL	36688	777-7777	S/N	Moderate	BTE100	Jul 7 85
Wellington, Biff	1 Porter House	Steak Island	AL	36661	999-9999	S/N	Moderate	ITE100	Sep 9 85
Xenia, Phoebe	414 Scary Lane	Spook City	AL	36679	000-0000	Mixed	Moderate	ITE100	Oct 10 85

Figure 14. Sort of hearing aid evaluation database for BTE and ITE fitting.

77

File: H. Aid Database
Report: 1st half/1985
Selection: Date Fitted is before Jul 1 85

Name	Address	City	State	Zip	Telephone	Loss-Type	Loss-Degree	Hrng Aid	Date Fitted
Atkins, Maudie	100 New Lane	Centerville	AL	36666	111-1111	S/N	Moderate	BTE100	Jan 1 85
Barlow, Homer	Newton Road	Newburgh	AL	36600	222-2222	S/N	Severe	BA100	Feb 2 85
Cuthbert, Calvin	200 North Road	Fishtown	AL	33660	333-3333	Mixed	Moderate	BTE100	Mar 3 85
Horton, Maxine	400 Happy Acres	Water Port	AL	36030	555-5555	Mixed	Moderate	ITE100	May 5 85
Lawrence, Warren	505 Grand Blvd.	View City	AL	36699	666-6666	Conductive	Moderate	BTE100	Jun 6 85

Figure 15. Sort of hearing aid evaluation database for persons fitted with a hearing aid before July 1, 1985.

that any clinic would have in the files. However, with the computerized database, the retrieval of the information is so much more efficient that there is a tendency to look more carefully at what has been done. (Imagine asking the secretary of a busy clinic to find all files of people seen between July 1 and September 1 who had moderate hearing losses and who had not been fitted with hearing aids.)

The fact that the information is so readily available promotes the use of it in developing a perspective on how the clinic works. Being able to see what has been done, when and how it was done, and perhaps by whom, can lead to an understanding of the clinic functions, which in turn can lead to improved decision making in developing clinic operations.

COMMERCIALLY AVAILABLE SOFTWARE FOR THE OFFICE

For individuals who are responsible for the business operation of a clinic, there are several commercially available programs which can increase office efficiency. Many programs for general ledger, accounts payable, accounts receivable, and inventory are available. These programs generally have enough flexibility that they can be adapted for almost any individual setting.

One of the most beneficial computer programs can be one for billing. Billing by hand is a time-consuming process for a busy clinic. Preparing the billing for mailing each month becomes a major chore that consumes the time of the office staff and thereby disrupts the normal office procedures. Computerized billing programs reduce the time significantly, and the more efficient the billing procedures, the less the time delay in billing and the more stable the clinic's funding. This is especially important for those in private practice and for those who administer clinics that must be self-supporting.

POTENTIAL USES

Case Load Analysis

In a time in which economics plays a critical role in whether agencies will flourish or fail, there is a great need for administrative efficiency. The administrator needs to be able to analyze the case load and relate it to amount of income generated. No speech and hearing clinic would restrict services solely on how much funding is generated by a particular service. However, services which lose money must be offset by those which generate funds.

Setting fees for services is difficult at best. One of the most commonly employed strategies is to simply raise fees across the board. While this is relatively easily defended, clinics would do well to analyze how much it is costing them to provide different services. If a clinic raises all fees, but then increases case load areas that do not generate as much money as other areas, it may find a budget shortfall at the end of the year.

Attendance

Another area in which clinics need information is attendance. Clinic directors who have analyzed client attendance records realize that the "no show" client represents a loss in both revenue and clinician time. Computer programs could be developed which would analyze attendance records to determine the effect of the various variables on attendance. Knowing the effects of scheduling on attendance by age, type of problem, day of the week, time of day, assigned clinician, type of treatment, etc. could lead to scheduling techniques which could reduce the amount of absenteeism.

Trend Analysis

Every clinic must be able to project needs. One of the best ways of determining what will be needed is to analyze changes in case load. By reviewing case loads over a period of years, the administrator can see changes and from those changes predict what the needs will be in the future.

CONCLUSION

As society in general moves forward into the information age, professions will find it necessary to have means of obtaining, processing, and interpreting data. The computer does not change the data, nor determine what changes will be needed in a profession. It is merely a vehicle which permits the accumulation and organization of data on a scale that has never been possible before. Agencies which develop the skill to use information databases will enter into the age with commensurate advantages. Those who do not develop the skill will be faced with a major challenge.

References

Bonner, P. (1983). It's all about time. *Personal Computing*, 7, 110–115, 218.
Foster, E. (1985). Building simple spreadsheets. *Personal Computing*, 9, 61–67.

Gabel, D. (1984). How to buy data-base software. *Personal Computing* **8,** 116–125, 206–209.

Heintz, C. (1984). To integrate or not to integrate. *Interface Age,* **9,** 76–81, 130–138.

Hood, S., & Miller, L. (1984). Administrative applications for microcomputers. In A. Schwartz (Ed.), *Handbook of microcomputer applications in communication disorders* (pp. 219–245). San Diego: College-Hill Press.

Krajewski, R. (1984). Database types. *Byte,* **9,** 137–150.

Lesk, M. (1984). Computer software for information management. *Scientific American,* **251,** 162–173.

McCarthy, M. (1984). Getting the most out of your spreadsheet. *Personal Computing,* **8,** 136–149.

Trost, S. (1982). *Doing business with VisiCalc.* Berkeley, CA: Sybex.

Wirth, N. (1984). Data structures and algorithms. *Scientific American,* **251,** 60–69.

Zarley, C. (1983). Dialing into data bases. *Personal Computing,* **7,** 135–139, 234.

7

The Computer in Speech–Language Pathology: A Review of the Literature

INTRODUCTION

The purpose of this chapter is to give the reader a perspective as to "where we are" and "how we got here" in regard to using computers in speech and language pathology. Most of the programs discussed in this chapter are not available to users in finished form. Some that are available have limited application because they were developed on mainframe computers that are not commonly available or they were written in computer languages that are not readily compatible with different operating systems. This chapter will give the reader an appreciation for the range of uses—clinical, administrative, and in other activities—for which members of the communication disorders community have found computer uses. The author feels that this type of perspective is necessary for the reader to understand and appreciate the current state of the art.

A review of the literature on computer utilization in communication disorders is, overall, an experience that is reassuring to the professional in the field. From the beginning, computer utilization in communication disorders has been marked by a satisfying blend of creativity and common sense. This has been due, in large measure, to the fact that the developments have been initiated by people within the field. The field of education has been criticized widely (Osgood, 1984) for the generally poor quality of the educational software that currently exists in the marketplace. Much of it was the result of software developed by computer programmers who knew a great deal about computers, but very little about the learning process.

An example of the problems in early educational software is found in the drill and practice type of programs. Since the drill and practice type of exercise is a natural for computer adaptation, it was not surprising that most of the programs took that form initially. Feedback paradigms for signalling the user when the response was right and wrong were usually included in the programs, but they lacked an understanding of what it takes to maintain motivation and interest in an activity.

Typically the program included some attention-getting graphic display when a correct response was made. Often, however, an equally attention-getting graphic was provided when a wrong response was achieved, thereby motivating students to make a wrong response occasionally just to see that graphic. Programs that rely on graphics are subject to saturation quickly. To get an idea of how long a child will maintain attention on a task involving graphic feedback, witness what happens with the commercially available video games (such as for the popular Atari) that include very professional graphics. There is an initial novel period during which the child will spend hours on the game. However, after a few sessions over a period of days the child usually tires of it. This can be attested to by those parents (author included) who can point to the stacks of commercially available games now residing in the closet.

Although the field of communication disorders has its fair share of drill and practice exercises, the range of uses to which the computer has been applied reflects the range of interests in the field itself. Much is to be learned from considering the processes that accompanied the early efforts. The following discussion of the early programs will include an account of what has been learned about using computers in the field.

EARLY PROGRAMS

Clinical Management

One of the earliest uses of the computer in communication disorders was an application to clinic management. Stunden (1966) reported on the development of a program at Western Michigan University which, in essence, matched clinicians and clients in the treatment process. The Speech Clinic had the task of creating schedules for 70–80 clients each semester.

The matching process was based on the parameters of time and space, client needs, and clinician needs.

The most critical parameter in the scheduling process is time because it involves finding times during which the client, clinician (and in some cases teams of clinicians and observers), and the supervisor are all free. However, time alone cannot dictate a schedule. Client needs, even in a training institution, are of paramount importance. The variables that must be considered before assigning a case to a clinician include general proficiency of clinician, academic preparedness, age and sex, and previous experience with type of case. The clinician's needs in terms of clock hours in the various disorder classifications and the need for experience with different ages and types of clients also must be considered.

If 10 or less clinicians are involved, the task of assigning cases can be accomplished with relative ease by simply meeting with the students. As the number of clinicians grows, however, the scheduling problems become increasingly complex. Considering the above variables, scheduling 50 students means consideration of thousands of possible combinations of clinician–client matches. The task that Stunden undertook was to reduce a job which consumed 70 hours of professional time for the clinic staff down to a more manageable chore.

In looking at this report, which was a pilot program, it is interesting to note that the first challenge they encountered was that of specifying the task, that is, identifying the variables and determining the procedure for achieving the goals. This is probably one of the most valuable outcomes of using computers. Programming requires that each task be described completely in symbolic representations that the computer can process. This dictates that the programmer consider carefully and thoroughly the parameters of the event for which a program is being developed. Those who have programmed will agree that working with the computer has the beneficial effect of requiring the user to think in logical, symbolic terms.

Record Keeping

One of the greatest strengths of the computer is its capacity for retaining large amounts of information. Creating, storing, and retrieving information are critical to almost all phases of a clinical or administrative operation.

In 1984 the author heard a presentation from members of a large metropolitan school system, which described how they had contracted with an accounting firm to develop a record keeping system for their children in special programs. The impetus for the project was the fact that the school system had several lawsuits against it for not having records on services for many of the children and many student records had been found to be incomplete and inaccurate. The cost of the new computer-managed record keeping system was over a $1 million and it had taken 4 years to implement it.

The school could have fared better by taking action earlier—and by keeping track of what was already happening in the field. Thirteen years prior to this project, Elliott, Vegely, and Falvey (1971) described an excellent approach to student record keeping. The basic goal of the system (entitled CORKS: *Computer-Oriented Record-Keeping System*) was to keep school and clinic records in the computer for fast and easy access and processing. Before writing the computer program, the authors astutely created a philosophical framework to guide the development of the program. Among the principles concerning the computer system were that it (1) should be easy to operate; (2) should store data in the smallest meaningful unit; (3) should be fitted to meet users' needs; (4) should be flexible; and (5) should have built-in quality control measures.

The report provides examples of data acquisition sheets, which are excellent models for any program. In fact, the report provides an excellent overall model that any organization or agency seeking to computerize its records could emulate. Among the advantages of CORKS was listed the following:

> Without question, we feel that the strongest immediate advantage of CORKS is related, not to its computer orientation, but to the fact that data judged as important and needed are systematically and completely collected at the point of origin. (Elliott *et al.*, 1971, p. 441)

In other words, it is often not the computer itself that brings the biggest change; it is the fact that working with the computer forces the user into acting on data in a consistent, systematic fashion.

Competency Evaluation

As third-party funding has become integrated into the financial network of the profession, a need has grown for greater accountability of services. When the PSROs (professional standards review organizations) were implemented. ASHA officials sought models for clinicians to consider. One such model was based on a computer review of services. Curlee (1973) published a report of the New Mexico Foundation for Medical Care, a PSRO designed to review Medicaid claims more efficiently. The Foundation enlisted the help of physicians to set guidelines for different diagnoses, including such variables as number of visits, laboratory tests, X rays, and therapy. These were compiled and programmed into the computer as was information concerning providers and patients. All claims filed were processed by the computer to ensure that the information on the claim was appropriate (for example, the name of the provider and the provider number matched). The computer then performed a routine check to determine if the claim was within the parameters defined in the guidelines. While all decisions were reviewed by professionals, the time required for review and the accuracy of the computer review greatly enhanced the efficiency of the review process.

Concerning the need for accountability procedures, Curlee (1973) suggested

> We must become willing to subject the services we provide the communicatively handicapped to the scrutiny of our professional peers. We must develop the competencies necessary to review the patterns of service provided by other speech pathologists and audiologists in a critical, professionally objective manner. (p. 417)

As the field becomes more accountable for its services, it will be increasingly important to maintain records of the results of treatment. It is the author's impression that as a profession, speech pathology provides services which are much more effective and efficient than client records indicate. Therefore, one goal of any clinical services program should be to develop data acquisition procedures that accurately reflect the effectiveness of the diagnostic and treatment practices. The computer, as a tool which requires logical, consistent data input, can be the vehicle through which this is achieved.

Clinic Operation

An example of how an individual clinic can achieve computer-assisted records is contained in a report by Kamara and Kamara (1976). This report describes the efforts of the Southeastern Ohio Hearing and Speech Center to computerize record-keeping procedures. The need to devise such a system was stated as follows:

> There is no question that all agencies must be accountable for the expediency, effectiveness, and cost of their service delivery system. The need is to find a system of internal financial and service analysis that will answer the greatest number of operational questions with the least amount of procedural effort. Inherent within this need is a cross-referencing of service information and cost factors to provide dynamic appraisal records. (Kamara & Kamara, 1976, p. 229)

Initially the goal was to develop a limited format to collect and retrieve data related to a grant. However, this was expanded to include information concerning the client such as primary disorder, reason for absences, referral status, type of service provided, length of treatment, and other information. Among the uses of the information, Kamara and Kamara (1976) reported:

Analysis of attendance which has led to a 16 percent improvement.
Grant requests specifying percent of activity in each community the agency serves as well as a detailed description (in tables) of the nature of the activity and the ages of the people receiving assistance (yielding approximately $50,000).
Growth analysis and future planning.
Certification statistics.
Board reports.
Summarized intraagency communication of activities presented and analyzed monthly, quarterly, and yearly. (p. 231)

As with the reports mentioned before, the system devised was based on a thorough, well-thought-out plan before the computer component was implemented. This report bears reading by any agency looking to computerize operations since it discusses the planning and commitment that must accompany such an effort.

Certification Records

One of the first record-keeping tasks for which the computer was used in the field of communication disorders was that of certification records. All speech–language pathologists and audiologists are aware of the need to maintain complete and accurate records of academic and clinical experiences. These are necessary to substantiate applications for the American Speech–Language–Hearing Association's Certificate of Clinical Competence. The first report was filed by Mahaffey (1973) in which he described the record-keeping procedures implemented at the University of Southern Mississippi. Each quarter the student entered information concerning courses and clinical experiences completed. The computer then calculated the totals and provided a listing of completed requirements and requirements yet to be met. This guided the student and advisor in scheduling academic and clinical experiences.

Peterson (1977) reported a similar system that increased input efficiency by having students record the data on optic-scan computer forms. Peterson reported that as a part of their data, students included information relative to evaluation. The training program at the University of Tennessee at that time included 35 possible supervisors and over 175 students, resulting in the need to process over 500 evaluation forms per quarter. Use of the computer made it possible to process this data in a more efficient manner.

Harlan and Hasegawa (1976) reported the development of computerized student records for certification at Purdue University. Their system was predicated on key punching data cards which, by current standards, would be awkward. Of import in the Harlan and Hasegawa study was the mention that students requested copies of printouts to send to prospective employers. In discussions with students, employers, and program directors, the author has found a consensus that computer printouts project a credibility that cannot be matched by a form containing the same information. In other words, information that is known to have been generated from a computer generally has a higher degree of credibility than information generated from a human.

One director of a sizable training program reported that when requests for documentation of clinical experiences are requested for state licensing and certifying agencies, he sends a computer printout of the information rather than having the student or a clerical person complete the forms sent by the state. He indicated that to that time no state had rejected the printout even though it was not in the format of their own forms. However, it has been reported that at least one state still requires information to be recorded on their own form.

The author has found the credibility of the computer to be outstanding. At one time he was working with a colleague in a service delivery consultancy which involved the submission of numerous reports. After a time it was decided that equipment should be upgraded from a dot matrix printer to a letter-quality printer. However, it was found that the computer reports generated on the letter-quality printer did not have as much credibility because they looked like they had been typed on a typewriter (that is, prepared by "human hand"). To restore the credibility of computer-generated processing, use of the dot matrix printer was reinstated.

A 1977 report of the computerization of records at Texas Christian University followed basically the same format of those reported above (Harden, Harden, & Norris, 1977). However, the information kept was extended to include factors which could be of value in program planning. Methods of treatment used with a case were recorded as well as the amount of time spent using the method. The number and type of supervisory activities performed by the clinic faculty were also recorded. Information related to clients included the types of treatment procedures used, the progress made using that treatment procedure, length of contact with the clinic, amount of time in treatment, and other factors.

Program analysis was accomplished by a series of sort programs which provided information such as clinicians supervised by each supervisor with total hours accumulated; and a record of student experiences, including type of disorder, age, treatment used, and results. The report indicated that posttreatment analysis was used to determine the effectiveness of different types of treatment approaches, including follow-up on the status of former clients, analysis of referral source, distribution of case load by disorder, age, and sex, and an analyis of the average length of treatment for various types of disorders. This type of information could be extremely important in planning for the future.

Computer-Assisted Clinical Management Analysis

In 1979, Oratio reported on the use of the computer as a means of analyzing clinical interaction. Using his protocol, an observer recorded interactions between the clinician and client. The critical variable in this paradigm was the sequence of interaction. Oratio pointed out that the analysis of a 20-item protocol sheet for two sequence patterns would require a search of 400 patterns (20 × 20). Taking it further, the analysis for three sequence interaction patterns would require search for 8000 (20 × 20 × 20) patterns.

He suggested that the analysis process could be reduced significantly by coding the information and programming the computer to identify the patterns. In the process, an observer initially coded all of the interactions according to the appropriate category (20 categories, 10 involving clinician behavior and 10 involving client behavior). This information was coded to the computer which ran searches and yielded information concerning number, percentages, and frequency of all possible two-, three-, and four-sequence patterns.

Although somewhat involved, the analysis yielded a moment by moment account of the clinical interaction. This would provide a supervisor with an abundance of discrete data which could be used in counseling clinicians. It also provides a consistent, systematic analysis of the clinical interaction process, with relatively objective information, which could be of value in research concerning the clinical interactive process.

An important point to be learned from this report was the strength of the computer in analyzing large amounts of data. It has been suggested that interaction that takes place in the clinical setting is too complex to break down into meaningful variables. While this may be true of analysis of interaction based on human processing, the computer has the potential to receive, store, and integrate data concerning clinical interaction that will provide data on many more aspects of the clinical process. This should lead to a better understanding of the clinical process and result in better training for clinicians.

EARLY CLINICAL APPLICATIONS

At the ASHA conventions in 1974 and 1975, the author presented information on the clinical applications of computers to communication disorders (Fitch & Terrio, 1974, 1975) At one meeting which had perhaps 50 people in attendance (in a room with a capacity of 500), there was polite applause at the end of the presentation. When the person who applauded approached him after the meeting, it was assumed that a convert had been made. However, the distinguished looking lady patted the author kindly on the shoulder and said, "that was real nice sonny, but computers will never get out of the laboratory." For a few years it seemed that she might be right, but it has been gratifying to see the field begin to view technology as a clinical entity and embrace its use.

The study presented in 1975 (Fitch & Terrio) described a laboratory arrangement whereby the computer acted as a decision maker and management of the treatment process. The client (test case was an 8-year-old girl) sat in a sound-treated room with a microphone and a monitor in front of her. The monitor was actually an oscilloscope on which dots could be arranged to make letters and words. The stimulus (sound, word, sentence) was printed on the monitor and the child spoke it. The signal received by the microphone was processed by a combination of filters, attenuators, and voice-activated relays that were programmed to determine whether or not the acoustic spectrum was appropriate for an /s/ phoneme. The child had a lisp but had been taught, and was capable of producing, a correct /s/ sound.

When the child produced the correct sound (i.e., when the equipment detected the presence of a target acoustic spectrum), a signal was sent to the computer. A reinforcing word (good!, great!, etc.) was printed on the monitor and the next stimulus was presented. The computer was programmed to present stimuli at a predetermined pace. If the child slowed below that pace, the computer ignored the item and presented the next stimulus. The computer was programmed with criteria to determine when to present more difficult stimuli (if the child was having a high success rate) and when to present less difficult material (when the child's success rate dropped). The clinician simply set up the equipment and then watched as the treatment session proceeded. (It should be noted, however, that the clinician talked with the child before and after the session to provide the human touch to treatment.)

The equipment involved was relatively sophisticated, and the time to program the apparatus excessive. However, it posed the answer to many of the problems of treatment administered by humans. First, computers do not have good days and bad days as do clinicians. The criteria are always the same so the day-to-day demands of treatment are consistent. Second, the computer is "all business"; it cannot be distracted by conversation from the patient. This results in the treatment session moving quickly. Third, the computer stores all the data concerning the session for later retrieval and analysis. By the computer doing the routine aspects of treatment, clinicians have more time to do the things that the computer cannot do, such as counseling.

In 1978, Fields and Renshaw presented a paper in which the computer was used to analyze a transciption of spontaneous speech. The purpose of the study was to determine if the computer could differentiate normal and language-disordered children through the analysis of the use of nouns and verbs. The findings in that study were that the computer method was no more efficient than traditional methods. However, it offered the suggestion that improved methods might reduce the amount of the professional's time involvement in the process.

The ability of the computer to analyze and organize data caught the attention of developers early in the history of computer applications. Sommers (1979) described a computerized analysis of the Edinburgh Articulation Test. The results were entered into the computer, which provided a comparison of the test stimulus and actual response and yielded a statistical feature analysis.

Telage (1980) used data from the McDonald Deep Test to achieve basically the same goal. The examiner entered errors in the computer from the keyboard in the form of initial/final sounds that could be recorded as substitutions and omissions. The computer was programmed to analyze the errors and provide printouts of error patterns by sound and by distinctive feature. The features were derived from those used by McReynolds and Engmann (1975), which were based on the Chomsky and Halle (1968) feature system. The results were several tables listing the errors by number and percentage.

In both of the analysis programs described above, existing diagnostic protocols were used and the computer was employed as an analysis device after the fact, that is, after the test was completed. While there is little doubt that the computer saved time in analyzing the results of the test, the time saved in analysis was offset by the time used in entering data into the computer from the test sheet. This requires considerable time which clinicians in the field would not find practical.

THE EMERGENCE OF THE COMPUTER-BASED CLINICIAN: THE PIONEERS

The 1980s marked the beginning of a new era in the field of communication disorders. Actually, the first formal events to bring attention to the potential of the computer occurred at the 1980 ASHA Convention. At that meeting, five of the scientific exhibits featured applications of microcomputers. The exhibits were very popular and observers were impressed by the attention paid the exhibits by practicing clinicians. At that convention there were only a few other computers being displayed in any capacity.

At the following convention, the ASHA Convention in Toronto in 1980, the response to the new technology was even greater. It marked the turning point in that there was no doubt in anyone's mind that computers were destined to be part of the clinical scene. Two of the best attended short courses were on computer applications (Mahaffey, 1981; Wilson & Fox, 1981a). Mahaffey impressed his audience with the potential of the computer for use in a wide range of activities and Wilson impressed them with a display of moving, talking computer animation.

At that convention the author chaired a double miniseminar on computers (Fitch, 1981a, b). The first was on clinical applications and the second on administrative applications. Whereas programs on computer applications at previous conventions had few attendees, the rooms in which these meetings were held were overflowing. At the end of the session, a crowd of people asking for information gathered around the participants. All handouts were given out and within 5 minutes 166 people had left their names and addresses to request more information.

Also at the ASHA convention in Toronto, the first organizational meeting for a computer users group was held. Russ Mills of the Ann Arbor Veteran's Administration Medical Center and Mike Rolnick of William Beaumont Hospital in Royal Oak, Michigan, were the driving force in that meeting. Their "crusade" began when a paper they had submitted to the program committee on computers was rejected. They protested to the program chairman, indicating that they felt there were many people in the field who wanted to hear more about computers. The program chairman provided them with a room for an evening to present their information.

Drs. Mills and Rolnick brought two computers, expecting to register those who came and then demonstrate some uses of the computer. The response to the session was so great, however, that the entire evening was spent just registering people. A short meeting was held to determine what to do next. Out of that meeting grew the impetus for the formation of CUSH (Computer Users in Speech and Hearing).

The people who initiated the push for computer applications were, to an extent, mavericks. They took technology and put it in the clinic room. While others had done this previously with various forms of technology on a limited basis, those associated with computers did it with an evangelistic fervor and commitment that frightened some.

The author was chairman of the ASHA Committee on Educational Technology during this time and received countless inquiries from clinicians in the field wondering what to do about the computer revolution. The overall tone of the inquiries was one of restrained panic. The question most often heard was "will the computer replace me?"

The pioneers, persons such as Carol Cohen, Bernie Fox and Mary Wilson, Rich Katz, Russ Mills, Mike Palin and Dennis Mordecai, Mike Rolnick, Gary Rushakoff and Marlo Schuldt, did not stop at evangelism. They were unlike any people that the field had seen before. Prior to this time, technological developments came out of a laboratory, were developed by a researcher, and, if they showed promise, entered the marketplace through an existing company.

There were no software companies for speech and hearing when the pioneers developed their programs, so they started the companies themselves. Only a person who knows how much time and effort that programming requires, and the time and financial resources that are needed to start such an operation, can realize that embarking on such an endeavor was not something that had been a part of the training of any one of them. They were truly entrepreneurs. It was their faith in their products that moved the field.

Although there was never doubt on the part of the pioneers, there was doubt as to how the field itself would react to members who marketed goods as well as services. The history of ASHA had been blotted by the ban on audiologists selling hearing aids. The inverted thinking of earlier years that profit would distort quality of service lingered in the minds of many. However, the powers that be in the profession applauded the entrepreneurial spirit of the software developers and became prime movers themselves in the push to incorporate technology into clinical activity. Fred Minifie was perhaps the most vocal as a representative of ASHA, and his presence and judgment were critical factors in acceptance by the field. Frank Kleffner and Ron Goldman were instrumental in recognizing the need for the field to move into computer utilization and took action within the American Speech–Language–Hearing Foundation to promote computer literacy and competency.

Today the pioneers are no longer pioneers. They are successful, established professionals and business persons who have carved a niche for themselves in the scheme of communication disorders. They have gained recognition and financial reward, and are leaders in the field. They represent models of success that may be instrumental in recruiting and maintaining in the field bright young individuals who are looking for a profession with outstanding opportunities.

INVOLVEMENT OF COMMERCIAL PUBLISHERS

When it became evident that computers would become an integral part of the clinical scene, companies that published clinical materials began developing expertise and organizational plans that included software components. The young professional today who develops a competent, useful computer program will find a host of opportunities to market his product. The publishers wisely chose to work with professionals in the field rather than hire programmers and develop their own products. They now have their own programmers, but the task of the publishing company programmer is to work with the professionals who develop programs to improve the technical efficiency of the product.

AN ORGANIZATION FOR PROFESSIONALS USING COMPUTERS

In 1982, CUSH (Computer Users in Speech and Hearing) was formed by a small group of interested professionals. The organization published quarterly newsletters in 1983 and 1984 and adopted a journal format in 1985. As of this writing, CUSH has approximately 800 members representing five different countries.

CONCLUSION

The field of communication disorders has been fortunate to have the right mixture of professional involvement, support from the professional association, and involvement of materials publishers in the initial stages of software development. If the trend continues, the profession will find itself among the leaders in service providers in the behavioral sciences.

References

Chomsky, N., & Halle, M. (1968). *The sound patterns of English.* New York: Harper & Row.

Curlee, R. (1973). New Mexico Foundation for Medical Care—A computer-assisted professional standard review organization. *Asha, 15,* 415–417.

Durkee, D. (1982). Maple sugar and apples: A yummy way to learn. *Softalk, 2,* 170–172.

Elliott, L., Vegely, A., & Falvey, N. (1971). Description of a computer oriented record-keeping system. *Asha, 13,* 435–443.

Fields, T. & Renshaw, S. (1978). *Use of the computer in the diagnosis of language disorders.* Paper presented to the American Speech and Hearing Association Annual Convention, San Francisco.

Fitch, J. (1981a). *The computer and speech and hearing services: Administrative applications.* Miniseminar presented to the American Speech–Language–Hearing Association Annual Convention, Toronto.

Fitch, J. (1982b). *The computer and speech and hearing services: Clinical applications.* Miniseminar presented to the American Speech–Language–Hearing Association Annual Convention, Toronto.

Fitch, J. (Ed.) (1982c). *Software Registry Number One.* American Speech–Language–Hearing Association, Committee on Educational Technology.

Fitch, J. (Ed.) (1982d). *Software Registry Number Two.* American Speech–Language–Hearing Association, Committee on Educational Technology.

Fitch, J., & Cross, S. (1983). Telecomputer treatment of aphasia. *Journal Speech and Hearing Disorders, 48,* 335–336.

Fitch, J., Davis, D., Evans, W., & Sellers, D. (1983). Computer managed screening for communication disorders. *Language, Speech, and Hearing Services in Schools, 15,* 66–69.

Fitch, J., & Terrio, L. (1974). *Computer-assisted programmed articulation therapy.* Paper presented to the American Speech and Hearing Association Annual Convention, Las Vegas.

Fitch, J. & Terrio, L. (1975). *Computer-assisted therapy for communication disorders.* Paper presented to the American Speech and Hearing Association Annual Convention, Washington, DC.

Gleason, G. (1981). Microcomputers in education: The state of the art. *Educational Technology, 21,* 7–18.

Harden, R. J., Harden, R. W., & Norris, M. (1977). Computer program for the analysis of clinical enrollment. *Asha, 19,* 472–474.

Harlan, N., & Hasegawa, A. (1976). Computer processing of graduate student clinical clock hours. *Asha, 18,* 295–298.

Kamara, C., & Kamara, A. (1976). Computer billing, service analysis, and financial reporting in a hearing and speech agency. *Asha, 18,* 229–231.

Mahaffey, R. (1973). A computerized procedure for keeping student records for ASHA-CCC requirements. *Asha, 15,* 590.

Mahaffey, R. (1981). *Strategies for using the digital computer in adult education.* Short course presented to the American Speech-Language-Hearing Association Annual Convention Los Angeles.

McReynolds, L., & Engmann, D. (1975). *Distinctive features analysis of misarticulations.* Baltimore: University Park Press.

Mills, R., & Thomas, R. (1981). Microcomputerized language therapy for the aphasic patient. In *Proceedings of the Johns Hopkins first national search for applications of personal computing to aid the handicapped* (pp. 45–46). Los Angeles: IEEE Computer Society Press.

Minifie, F. (1981). Graduate education during a technological revolution. *National Council of Graduate Programs in Speech and Language Pathology and Audiology Proceedings* (pp. 1–9).

Oratio, A. (1979). Computer-assisted interaction analysis in speech–language pathology and audiology. *Asha, 21,* 179–184.

Osgood, D. (1984). A computer on every desk. *Byte, 9,* 162–184.

Peterson, H. (1977). More about computer-assisted clinical record keeping. *Asha, 19,* 617–618.

Rushakoff, G. (1982). *Design and implementation of a course in clinical microcomputer applications for speech–language pathologists and audiologists.* Unpublished doctoral dissertation, University of Florida.

Rushakoff, G., & Lombardino, L. (1983). Comprehensive microcomputer applications for non-vocal, severely physically handicapped children. *Teaching Exceptional Children, 16,* 18–22.

Rushakoff, G., Vinson, B., Penner, K., & Messal, S. (1979). *Clinical decision making through electronic information processing.* Paper presented to the American Speech–Language–Hearing Association Annual Convention, Atlanta.

Seron, X., Deloche, G., Mouland, G., & Rousselle, M. (1980). A computer-based therapy for the treatment of aphasic subjects with writing disorders. *Journal of Speech and Hearing Disorders, 45,* 45–58.

Sommers, R. (1979). Using the computer to analyse articulation test data. *British Journal of Disorders of Communication, 14,* 231–240.

Stunden, A. (1966). Computer simulation of therapy—the client–clinician match. *Asha, 8,* 100–104.

Telage, K. (1980). A computerized plane-manner distinctive feature program for articulation analyses. *Journal of Speech and Hearing Disorders, 45,* 481–493.

Wilson, M., & fox, B. (1980). *Computer approaches to language diagnosis and treatment in communication disorders.* Paper presented to the Region Ten Convention of the American Association of Mental Deficiency, Hartford, Connecticut.

Wilson, M., & Fox, B. (1981a). *Microcomputer courseware development: The challenge of the eighties.* Short course presented to the American Speech–Language–Hearing Association Annual Convention, Los Angeles.

Wilson, M., & Fox, B. (1981b). The bilingual computer: Promise of the eighties. *Asha, 23,* 651–652.

Wilson, M., & Fox, B. (1983). Microcomputers: A clinical aid. In H. Winitz (Ed.), *For Clinicians, by Clinicians* (pp. 235–248). Baltimore: University Park Press.

8

Speech–Language Pathology: Diagnosis

INTRODUCTION

It is redundant, but important, to restate that the clinician is still the critical element in the clinical process. By itself, the computer has nothing to offer diagnostically. But in the hands of the capable user, it can be a tool that will make evaluations faster, more efficient, and more accurate. For a discussion of diagnostic software to be meaningful, it is necessary to look carefully at the diagnostic process itself and conceptualize a meaningful model.

A Diagnostic Model

Since it is basically a problem-solving process, clinical diagnostic procedures should follow the steps of the scientific method. The dichotomy between clinical and research methodology is an artificial one that needs to be discarded (Schiefelbusch, 1980). The steps in the diagnostic process should include essentially the following: it should collect information, analyze information, formulate diagnosis, prescribe treatment based on diagnosis, and evaluate treatment to confirm validity of diagnosis.

As the use of the computer in the diagnostic process is analyzed in this chapter, reference will be made to the elements above. It follows that evaluation of programs by clinicians should be on the basis of whether a software package contains the elements suggested. The computerization of diagnostic procedures is still in its infancy and few software packages provide help in the execution of more than one of the elements.

Working toward the Model

Critics of computer software are quick to point out that developers are doing nothing innovative to the diagnostic or treatment process. They suggest that developers merely take existing material and put it into the computer. These critics suggest that developers should take advantage of the unique qualities of the computer to formulate new diagnostic or treatment strategies.

The author is in agreement with this critique of software for the field of communication disorders. However, the reader should be aware that there is probably a minimum delay of one generation between the emergence of any powerful new technology and its general acceptance. The potential that the computer possesses is far more advanced than anything that has been available in the past. The treatment and diagnostic strategies that people now working in the field are employing are those learned in their training programs. It will be years before training programs change, and then only will the utilization of the computer in the clinical process approach its potential.

What the field can expect is a predictable pattern of software development. Initially the computer will be used in conjunction with traditional tests. Data generated from the tests will be entered into the computer and the computer will perform analysis of selected features. The analysis will be output to the printer with comprehensive compilations of the behaviors assessed and patterns of errors noted.

The next step in software development will be the emergence of tests especially designed for direct input to the computer, thus eliminating, or at least substantially reducing, the role that the clinician now plays in collecting information for diagnosis. Initially, the method of collecting information will still require clinician mediation (a clinician will be involved in the data acquisition process), but later paradigms will be developed in which the computer can accept data directly.

The next step in development will be the inclusion of AI (artificial intelligence) in the software. Not only will the software analyze the patterns of behavior, and patterns of errors, but it will also formulate hypotheses concerning the etiology and maintaining conditions of the disorder. In this regard, the computer will suggest possible factors of origin and maintenance of the disorder and recommend further testing procedures to confirm or deny the hypotheses. In effect, the computer will be used to employ the concept of differential diagnosis.

The step beyond that will be computer software that, after all the information is acquired and analyzed, generates prescriptive treatment programs. Treatment programs (to be discussed in the next chapter) will contain accountability features that will input back to the computer data concerning the performance of the patient in treatment. If the treatment for a given patient is successful, and that treatment is based on the results of the diagnosis, it can be assumed that the diagnosis was correct. If not, corrections of diagnosis can be made based on that information.

It is difficult to envision how the computer is going to affect the clinical process in the future, other than to acknowledge the fact that it will indeed change it. The author hopes that those taking critical looks at the software being developed today keep in mind that the application of technology to its fullest potential takes time. If they can be generous in this regard, they can more fully appreciate the efforts of early developers.

ARTICULATION

The early programs in articulation diagnosis were developed on mainframe computers and required substantial time to prepare the data for computer analysis. One of the first, *CONSPAN,* required the clinician first to make a narrow transcription of a speech sample and then code the elements numerically (Faircloth & Faircloth, 1970). The computer program then made an exhaustive listing of the distinctive features and error patterns. While it was an excellent tool for training students, the excessive time required to code the information negated its use by the practicing clinician.

The work of Sommers (1979) and Telage (1980) represented efforts to adapt existing tests to computer analysis. Again, both were developed on mainframe computers. Sommers (1979) used the computer to analyze articulation performance data that was obtained from the administration of the Edinburgh Articulation Test. The computerized analysis was a comparison of the test items with the actual production of the sound and a statistical feature analysis.

Telage (1980) used the computer to perform a feature analysis of errors obtained using the McDonald Deep Test of Articulation (McDonald, 1964). The sounds tested were categorized according to features based on a modified version of the distinctive features system developed by Chomsky and Halle (1968). A system of binary coding was used to evaluate features.

A substitution error did not always result in a feature being in error. For example, if an error fricative were substituted for a target fricative, the fricative feature would not be in error. The system had the advantage of identifying significant error patterns according to feature.

A prophetic statement from that article reads as follows: "the current technical revolution in the microprocessor field is expected to place millions of highly versatile computers in homes within a few decades. If this occurs, such devices will undoubtedly become commonly used machines" (Telage, 1980, pp. 481–482). Substitute the "years" for "decades" and the prophecy is fulfilled.

None of the programs above were developed for general distribution. The first software packages which were developed for commercial distribution will be discussed in the next sections.

Lingquest I: Phonological Analysis

Lingquest I: Phonological Analysis, an analysis tool developed by Palin and Mordecai (1982), was one of the first to gain widespread attention. Word lists, or a spontaneous sample of up to 120 words, may be entered by the clinician using the program. Both the actual production and the idealized (model) production are entered. Data disks of the model production for the Photo Articulation Test (Pendergast, Dickey, Selmar, & Soder, 1969) and the Compton–Hutton Phonological Assessment (Compton & Hutton, 1978) have been entered on data disks for the users' convenience. Either narrow or broad transcriptions can be used. When the data has been entered, the computer performs a comparison of the actual production against the model production.

Profiles of errors are available for singleton and blend sounds as well as for omissions and substitutions. Vowel error analysis is included. The computer indicates the type of feature, the number of times that it was attempted, the number of times it was in error, and the percentage of error. The analysis is performed in a very short period of time and the printouts are comprehensive. The information helps the clinician to identify the underlying phonological structure and identify errors patterns. This reduces the amount of time spent in analyzing the data and maximizes the information that the clinician has to work with in planning treatment.

Computer-Aided Intelligibility Diagnosis

Computer-Aided Intelligibility Diagnosis (Yorkstron, Beukelman, & Traynor, 1984) is another example of adapting an existing device to computer analysis. The original test was a pencil and paper test with manual scoring. The premise for CAID is a simple one. An audio recording is made of the client reading (or repeating) words and sentences with known content. Judges then listen to the words and sentences and write down what they think the person said. What the judges report hearing is then compared to the original script. Intelligibility is measured by the percentage of words that were correctly identified by the judges.

The manual scoring of CAID was laborious. The computer scoring is much more efficient. The judges can enter the sentences directly into the computer so that no transition from pencil and paper to computer is needed. The records are maintained on diskette and results can be output to a printer.

A simple, straightforward program such as CAID can be a time-saving tool for clinicians who need to have records of client intelligibility. Not only aphasics, but laryngectomees and severe articulation cases as well can be evaluated using this tool.

Computer-Managed Articulation Diagnosis

The author developed a tool for articulation diagnosis based on compromise of various features of other tests and an attempt to make the most of computer capabilities (Fitch, 1985a). Before developing the *Computer-Managed Articulation Diagnosis* (CMAD), he had developed a screening test, a component of which evaluated articulation. (This will be discussed in a later section). In the initial attempt, he tried to adapt an existing test. The experience led him to understand that computer-based evaluation tools should be designed especially for computers. It is his belief now that, in most cases, adaptations of existing materials will not tap the full potential of the computer.

With this in mind, he developed CMAD from scratch, employing clinical biases developed from his own experiences. One such bias is that connected speech provides a more accurate environment for evaluating articulation. However, evaluating connected speech through analyzing spontaneous speech samples is exceedingly time consuming and often the samples of spontaneous speech do not contain all sounds.

As a compromise between the efficiency of single-word tests and the accuracy of connected speech samples, he chose to use an elicited sentence approach. The target phonemes are embedded in sentences that appear on the screen. Clients read the target, if they can read. If not, the clinician models the target and the client repeats the model. While no formal studies have been conducted to evaluate the difference between response modes, clinical experiences to data suggest that the individual with misarticulations in spontaneous connected speech will make the same errors in elicited connected speech. This is in agreement with findings in language that led to the development of elicited language tests such as the Northwestern Syntax Screening Test (Lee, 1971) and the Carrow Elicited Inventory (Carrow, 1974).

The sounds in CMAD are tested only in pre- and postvocalic positions. This is in agreement with articulatory dynamics as espoused by Stetson (1951) and McDonald (1964), who suggested that syllabic integrity is most accurately assessed by considering the releasing and arresting features of consonants.

The test is administered directly from the computer and client responses input directly to the computer, eliminating the need to transfer script to computer. Errors can be input as distortions, substitutions, and omissions, and distortions can be judged as mild, moderate, or severe. Substitutions can be standard sounds or codes developed by the user. Both individual sounds and blends can be assessed. The test also has a component for assessing stimulability of error sounds.

When the test is completed, the results can be stored on diskette and/ or printed out. Test results stored on diskette can be recalled and edited or printed when desired. The printout of results includes a breakdown of errors by traditional physiological distinctive features. Analysis of errors for manner of production, place of articulation, voicing, and prevocalic/ postvocalic syllabic integrity is also included. Figures 16–19 are examples of the reporting format.

A study of the use of the test by public school personnel indicated that the test requires about the same time to administer as other tests, but the analysis and reporting features of CMAD reduce the amount of time for analysis drastically and provide maximum information concerning error patterns of misarticulations (Taylor, 1984). In the same study, it was found that results agreed significantly with results of the Arizona Articulatory Proficiency Scale (Fudala, 1970), the Templin–Darley Test of Articulation (Templin & Darley, 1969), and the Goldman–Fristoe Test of Articulation (Goldman & Fristoe, 1972).

Other Articulation Analysis Programs

Other articulation analysis programs are the *BLACHE Phonemic Inventory* (BPI) (Blache, 1984) and Process Analysis by Computer (Weiner, 1982). The BPI provides several types of analyses of the articulation sample. It provides an estimate of the level of development, noting the first system that needs treatment, as well as a listing of defective sounds at each developmental level, a listing of the sounds that are most defective, and a listing of sounds that are borderline defective. In addition, the BPI

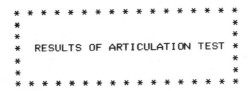

```
* * * * * * * * * * * * * * * * *
*                               *
*                               *
*    RESULTS OF ARTICULATION TEST *
*                               *
*                               *
* * * * * * * * * * * * * * * * *
```

NAME: MARTIN, KIM L..   DOB: 5/5/79   AGE: 5-1

SCHOOL/AGENCY: SPEECH/HEARING   DATE OF EVALUATION: 5/31/84

EXAMINER: JLF

	SOUND IN SENTENCE				SOUND IN BLEND		
	SOUND	PRE	POST	STIM	BLEND	PROD	STIM
1.	P				TW		
2.	B				KW		
3.	M		FR		PL	PW	EX
4.	H		FR		BL	BW	EX
5.	N				GL	GW	EX
6.	K	T	EX		KL	K-	EX
7.	G				FL	F-	EX
8.	W				SL	SW	EX
9.	F		P	GD	BR	BW	FR
10.	V	-	B	GD	PR	PW	FR
11.			N	EX	TR	TW	FR
12.	T				DR	DW	FR
13.	D				KR	K-	FR
14.	L	W	-	GD	GR	G-	FR
15.	Y				SM	-M	FR
16.	SH	CH	-	GD	SN	-N	FR
17.	CH		-	GD	SK	-K	FR
18.	J	D	-	FR	ST	-T	FR
19.	R	W	-	PR	SP	-P	FR
20.	S	TH1	-	FR	SKR	THKW	PR
21.	Z	D	-	FR	SPL	THP	PR
22.	TH1	T	-	PR	STR	THTW	PR
23.	TH2	D	-	PR	SPR	THPW	PR
24					SKW	THK	PR

COMMENTS:

KIM WAS COOPERATIVE DURING THE ENTIRE TEST.   HOWEVER-IT
WAS BROUGHT TO THE ATTENTION OF THE EXAMINER THAT KIM
HAD BEEN SICK THE DAY AND NIGHT BEFORE THE TEST.   THIS
COULD HAVE AFFECTED PERFORMANCE.

Figure 16.   Computer-managed articulation diagnosis—basic test data results.

```
          * * * * * * * * * * * * * * * *
          *                             *
          *    DISTINCTIVE FEATURES     *
          *                             *
          *         ANALYSIS            *
          *                             *
          *    PREVOCALIC POSITION      *
          *                             *
          * * * * * * * * * * * * * * * *
```

NAME: MARTIN, KIM L.   RECORD NUMBER: 4

AGE: 5 YEARS 1 MONTHS   DATE OF EVALUATION: 5/31/84

AGENCY: SPEECH/HEARING

	BILABIAL	LABIO DENTAL	LINGUA-DENTAL	LINGUA-ALVEOLAR	LINGUA-PALATAL	LINGUA-VELAR	GLOTTAL
	UNV VOC	UNV VOC	UNV VOC	UNV VOC	UNV VOC	UNV VOC	UNV VOC
PLOSIVES						T	
FRICATIVES		−	T D	TH1 D	CH		
AFFRICATES						D	
NASALS							
GLIDES					W * W		

* = Y (VOICED)

Figure 17. Computer-managed articulation diagnosis—prevocalic error analysis.

```
          * * * * * * * * * * * * * * * *
          *                             *
          *    DISTINCTIVE FEATURES     *
          *                             *
          *         ANALYSIS            *
          *                             *
          *    POST VOCALIC POSITION    *
          *                             *
          * * * * * * * * * * * * * * * *
```

NAME: MARTIN, KIM L.   RECORD NUMBER: 4

AGE: 5 YEARS 1 MONTHS   DATE OF EVALUATION: 5/31/84

AGENCY: SPEECH/HEARING

	BILABIAL	LABIO DENTAL	LINGUA-DENTAL	LINGUA-ALVEOLAR	LINGUA-PALATAL	LINGUA-VELAR	GLOTTAL
	UNV VOC	UNV VOC	UNV VOC	UNV VOC	UNV VOC	UNV VOC	UNV VOC
PLOSIVES							
FRICATIVES		P B	− −	− −	−		
AFFRICATES					− −		
NASALS						N	
GLIDES				− −			

Figure 18. Computer-managed articulation diagnosis—postvocalic error analysis.

```
* * * * * * * * * * * * *
*                       *
*  ERROR ANALYSIS SHEET *
*                       *
*         PAGE 1        *
*                       *
* * * * * * * * * * * * *
```

NAME; MARTIN, KIM L.   DATE: 5/5/79

EXAMINER; JLF   SCHOOL/AGENCY: SPEECH/HEARING

            ERRORS/TOTAL   ERRORS/TOTAL

TOTAL   PLOSIVES

    DISTORTION   0/42   DISTORTION   0/12
    SUBSTITUTION   12/42   SUBSTITUTION   1/12
    OMISSION   10/42   OMISSION   0/12
    TOTAL   22/42   TOTAL   1/12

PREVOCALIC   FRICATIVES

    DISTORTION   0/22   DISTORTION   0/15
    SUBSTITUTION   9/22   SUBSTITUTION   7/15
    OMISSION   1/22   OMISSION   6/15
    TOTAL   10/22   TOTAL   13/15

POST VOCALIC   AFFRICATES

    DISTORTION   0/20   DISTORTION   0/ 4
    SUBSTITUTION   3/20   SUBSTITUTION   1/ 4
    OMISSION   9/20   OMISSION   2/ 4
    TOTAL   12/20   TOTAL   3/ 4

UNVOICED   NASALS

    DISTORTION   0/17   DISTORTION   0/ 5
    SUBSTITUTION   5/17   SUBSTITUTION   1/ 5
    OMISSION   4/17   OMISSION   0/ 5
    TOTAL   9/17   TOTAL   1/ 5

VOICED   GLIDES

    DISTORTION   0/25   DISTORTION   0/ 6
    SUBSTITUTION   7/25   SUBSTITUTION   2/ 6
    OMISSION   6/25   OMISSION   2/ 6
    TOTAL   13/25   TOTAL   4/ 6
```

**Figure 19.** Computer-managed articulation diagnosis—distinctive features analysis (two pages).
```

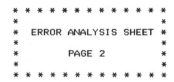

```
* * * * * * * * * * * * *
*                       *
*   ERROR ANALYSIS SHEET *
*                       *
*          PAGE 2       *
*                       *
* * * * * * * * * * * * *
```

NAME; MARTIN, KIM L.   DATE: 5/5/79

EXAMINER; JLF   SCHOOL/AGENCY: SPEECH/HEARING

              ERRORS/TOTAL   ERRORS/TOTAL

BILABIALS   LINGUA-PALATALS

    DISTORTION   0/ 7   DISTORTION   0/ 9
    SUBSTITUTION   0/ 7   SUBSTITUTION   3/ 9
    OMISSION   0/ 7   OMISSION   4/ 9
    TOTAL   0/ 7   TOTAL   7/ 9

LABIO-DENTALS   LINGUA-VELARS

    DISTORTION   0/ 4   DISTORTION   0/ 5
    SUBSTITUTION   2/ 4   SUBSTITUTION   2/ 5
    OMISSION   1/ 4   OMISSION   0/ 5
    TOTAL   3/ 4   TOTAL   2/ 5

LINGUA-DENTALS   GLOTTALS

    DISTORTION   0/ 4   DISTORTION   0/ 1
    SUBSTITUTION   2/ 4   SUBSTITUTION   0/ 1
    OMISSION   2/ 4   OMISSION   0/ 1
    TOTAL   4/ 4   TOTAL   0/ 1

LINGUA-ALVEOLARS

    DISTORTION   0/12
    SUBSTITUTION   3/12
    OMISSION   3/12
    TOTAL   6/12
```

**Figure 19.**  Continued

provides a breakdown of errors by place of articulation, manner of pro-
duction, and voicing. It can also provide a listing of the distinctive features
in need of treatment and an individualized listing of sound-pair contexts
for treatment.

A second program from Blache, the *Sound Substitution Analysis* pro-
gram (SSA) (1984), does an in-depth evaluation of the error pattern, in-
dicating the average number of distinctive features missed. This is an in-
dication of the severity of the articulation disorder. It also provides a
```

count of features missed on each substitution and indicates the error pattern. Both the BPI and the SSA have report features which provide rapid printouts of the results.

Weiner's *Process Analysis by Computer* (1982) analyzes transcriptions of 54 common words entered into the computer by using phonetic symbols. The misarticulations are then analyzed according to 24 phonological processes and misarticulations are listed by process. Summary of results tables are available and can be output to a printer.

NEEDS FOR ARTICULATION TESTS

A review of the tests above indicates that none comes close to tapping the full potential of the computer. Most use the computer to assist in only one phase of the diagnostic process, that of analysis of data. (All of the above utilize the computer in the collection of data, but it is only to the extent that the user enters information from the keyboard.) Although most of the tools provide breakdowns of error patterns, none actually formulate diagnosis. Some provide lists of stimuli which can be translated into treatment plans, but none generates specific plans or contains elements for checking validity of diagnosis. Remember that it is possible to do all these things with the computer; it just has not been done. In the following section, the needs for developing hardware and software will be discussed according to the elements involved.

Collecting Data

It is the author's belief that the greatest breakthrough in computer utilization for articulation diagnosis will occur when it can be used as the primary tool for collecting data or obtaining the articulation sample. The technology for doing so now exists and efforts are being made to bring the instrumentation to a clinically acceptable level of performance.

Obtaining a speech sample directly requires having the speaker talk into a transducer that changes the waves of sound pressure into electrical impulses that the computer can process. The means for doing this is called analog-to-digital (A/D) conversion. Basically, A/D works in the following manner. Sound strikes the microphone in constantly changing waves of air pressure. The microphone converts the physical signal of the movement of air particles into an electrical signal of the same relative magnitude. The electrical wave is then transmitted through wires to devices that process it in some manner. Common systems which process the wave include amplification of the wave (such as in public address systems), storing the wave (such as in tape recorders), and analyzing the wave (such as the sound spectrograph).

The A/D converter changes the wave into digital information which the computer can manipulate. It does so by sampling the sound wave at specified time intervals and recording the voltage present at each time. This results in passive data that can be analyzed in a number of different ways and reproduced for inspection at any time. A/D conversion was discussed earlier in Chapter 2 (Fig. 6).

A/D Conversion can be used in articulation testing by the fact that the process of A/D conversion permits a signal to be stored, so that models of correct production of sounds can be stored in the computer. Those models can be built on statistically based norms to ensure that they have maximum intelligibility to listeners who are representative of the general population. The model can be constructed by analyzing many speakers' productions of the sounds and making statistical prototypes. Thus, the model may be different from any single speaker.

Once the model is complete, clients' productions of sounds can be entered into the computer, stored, and compared to the models to determine statistical accuracy. The degree of error can be based on statistical comparison. The phrase *Within normal limits* for articulation ($\pm$ one standard deviation) can become a real, quantifiable concept.

The advantages of such a model for diagnosis are many. Primarily, it could truly standardize the articulation evaluation process. At the present time the validity and reliability of diagnostic articulation testing tools are dependent on the ability of the listener to make a judgment on a sound. Inter- and intrajudge reliability are difficult to ensure because the judges themselves are dynamic entities whose abilities and judgments change constantly. In a daily situation, perception by a judge may be dependent on the time of day (clinicians may make the best judgments early), order of sequence (judgments after working with severely disordered articulation cases may be different than ones made after working with clients with normal articulatory skills), and condition of the judge (judgments made when the judge does not feel well are not generally as accurate). Because humans are influenced by a large number of variables, the validity and reliability of judgments of articulatory behaviors are suspect.

Efforts to develop instruments to accomplish the above date back to the visible speech instrumentation (Potter, Kopp, & Green, 1947). The sound spectrograph was considered a breakthrough because it made all the parameters of the sound wave (frequency, intensity, and time) visible. However, the sound spectrograph was not found to be an effective tool for teaching articulatory proficiency. The patterns were too nebulous and complex to be overtly used to determine whether a sound was produced correctly or not. Furthermore, they were not quantifiable to the extent that norms could be specified. What the spectrograph did was make a visual picture of the acoustic event. Since the acoustic event itself is so fast moving and complex, simply reproducing it visually did nothing to simplify or quantify the signal.

Several efforts have been made in the area of providing speech aids for the deaf which simplified the information somewhat (Pickett, 1968), but these still did not find wide acceptance. One computer-based device that is working toward a resolution of the problem is the Video Voice (1984). In 1984 it was recognized as one of the 100 most significant technological advances by the editors of *Research and Development* magazine. The Video Voice, however, does not analyze articulation patterns of consonants per se. It is constructed to recognize components of formats one and two of vowels and present a visual representation of their relationship on the screen. However, it has an important feature that earlier instruments lacked. It formulates a percentage of the signal that is correct and this is registered on the screen. That is the key to effective instrumentation— reducing the decision to comparison of quantifiable data of the attempted sound to data of a model of that sound.

Other efforts to develop electronic devices to analyze speaking patterns are in development. One that the author has not viewed, but appears to hold promise, is the Computer-Aided Speech Production and Training (CASPT). Users can program models for the computer which it can compare to input from the client. Incorrect productions are not recognized by the computer, whereas correct production permits participation in a video game (Cooper & Nielson, 1984). Efforts at vowel recognition and specification will most likely be the first to bear fruit, because vowels are longer in duration and more stable from one phonemic environment to another. Computer recognition and comparison of sounds would not be subject to the same influences that affect human performances. For this reason alone, computer determination of speech sound integrity will represent a significant advance in the diagnosis of articulation.

Analyzing Data

The computer is already being utilized in the analysis of articulation and the paradigms now being employed are meaningful ones whose use would be continued, regardless of the means of collecting the sample. This appears to be the one area in which the field has made the strongest effort to date.

Formulating Diagnosis

The basic information concerning a diagnosis is critical to the selection of an appropriate treatment strategy. The basic elements of a diagnosis are as follows:

It confirms or denies the presence of a disorder.

It specifies the nature of the disorder (e.g., functional or organic).

It specifies the degree of impairment (e.g., mild, moderate, severe).

It suggests possible etiologies (e.g., imitated behavior, structural deviations).

It suggests the degree to which the disorder is amenable to treatment (i.e., the prognosis).

These basic elements are required if the clinician is to be able to interpret the findings of the evaluation to the client or the client's family in a meaningful way. They are also necessary in determining the treatment strategy to be employed. The decisions that contribute to the diagnosis are based on analysis of the information obtained. In most cases, the diagnosis is evident when the information is appropriately assembled.

The fact that diagnosis is based on logic makes it a task that is appropriate for the computer. Computers can be used to rapidly analyze the information in a myriad of ways that would require a substantial time commitment if completed by the clinician. The computer can also store statistical models to which the client's responses can be compared. From this, the computer can calculate the probability that a particular error pattern is related to certain disorders.

Furthermore, one can envision a diagnostic model that would analyze error patterns and project the three most likely etiologies, and even indicate the probability of accuracy of the diagnosis. While the clinician will still make the final decision, the routine analysis of data could be eliminated from the decision-making process. Significant efforts have not yet been directed to this area. The author feels that for the profession to increase credibility of its diagnostic efforts as a whole, it needs to utilize more quantifiable, statistical models. The computer can be important in accomplishing this goal.

Formulating Treatment Prescription

After conducting a clinical evaluation, the report is prepared, filed, and the client scheduled for treatment. Often the clinician assigned responsibility for treatment is not the one who completed the evaluation. After reading the report, the clinician is supposed to formulate an appropriate treatment plan.

The author suggests that just as the dichotomy between research and clinical activities is an artificial and inappropriate one, the separation of the diagnostic procedure from the treatment procedure is artificial and inappropriate. An integral part of a diagnostic procedure should be the development of a realistic, organized treatment plan. Clinicians completing the diagnosis should know the most about the client, and therefore, they should be in the best position to plan the treatment.

Developing treatment plans, like writing reports, is probably one of the least popular duties of a clinician. It is here again that the computer can play a meaningful role that will make life much more pleasant for the clinician. While this area has yet to be developed, it is suggested that it will be one of the most fruitful of areas to be explored.

One of the few models was proposed as early as 1981 (Schuldt, 1983). The system, entitled *Computerized Diagnostic and Treatment System* (CDTS), used the computer to lead the clinician through processes of logic that would lead to information needed for the treatment plan. The developer used the computer as an instrument to perform what amounted to differential diagnosis. The clinician entered information concerning the case to the computer. The computer analyzed the information and asked questions concerning the client. Each answer was analyzed and, depending on the response of the user, the computer selected the next question to ask. At the end of the branching process, the computer gave sources to which the user could refer for treatment ideas. The tangible end result was a specific reading list for treatment of the specific problem posed.

One can envision the day that the computer will do the above, but rather than simply provide references, it will generate several possible treatment plans from which the clinician can choose. The clinician, as usual, is the final authority as to what will be used. He is relieved, however, of the time-consuming task of collecting and collating existing treatment paradigms.

Validating Diagnostic Findings

This is an activity that will probably not gain attention until the other elements of the diagnostic process have been subjected to computer management by a variety of techniques. The author suggests that very few programs do validate diagnosis.

The question of how to determine whether a diagnosis was valid has not been resolved. The primary means of making the determination, however, can be done through a consideration of the accuracy of the diagnostic information. For example, if a diagnosis included prescriptive treatment that was appropriate for disorders with a similar diagnosis, and it was found that that treatment brought observable behavioral gains, it would be an indication that the diagnosis was correct. Another element that can be confirmed is the accuracy of the prognosis. Definitive prognoses that are found to be correct are strong indications of valid diagnoses.

The type of corroborative data that is needed to validate diagnosis on a continuing basis requires extensive records of treatment programs. If the results of treatment strategies for various disorders are stored, models can be built which validate the treatment programs themselves. Once treatment programs are standardized with known efficiency for known disorders, then results of individual treatment programs can be compared to the models. Positive agreement of results of an individual's treatment, and results of the same treatment for a diagnostic model, can then be used to validate individual diagnosis. This will be discussed more fully in the chapter on treatment (Chapter 9).

LANGUAGE

The diagnosis of language disorders does not have the history of study in the field of communication disorders that articulation has. Language is not as organized; anything and everything in communication *can* be put under the heading of language, including articulation, comprehension of spoken and written stimuli, expression of spoken and written stimuli, nonverbal communication, and so on. The efforts that have been made to use the computer in language diagnosis in the field of communication disorders to this point have been primarily concerned with the analysis element of the diagnostic process. However, some treatment strategies employing the computer (which will be discussed in the next chapter), particularly in the area of aphasia, often have baseline acquisition components or pretests that can be considered somewhat diagnostic in nature.

Transcription Analysis

One of the first widely used programs was *Lingquest I* (Mordecai, Palin, & Palmer, 1982). *Lingquest I* was developed along the same lines as *Lingquest II* (Palin & Mordecai, 1982). This program functions on the basis of the user entering a transcription of the actual spoken utterance into the computer, and then entering the correct (expanded) form of the utterance. The program analyzes the input to determine the number of occurrences of different language forms as well as the number and percentage of correct and incorrect usages. These are detailed in a report form that provides the user with a comprehensive analysis of the client's expressive language (Appendix C).

Miller and Chapman (1982) took a different approach in developing a computer-based language analysis called *Systematic Analysis of Language Transcripts* (SALT). Their protocol contained provisions for analyzing both interactional language between speakers and intrasubject language. The program provided measures of mean length of utterance (in morphemes and words), distribution of utterances (by morphemes and words), frequency of occurrence of words used, occurrence of bound morphemes, and frequency tables for word classes. It provides interactional analysis based on number and ratio of speaking events per speaker.

Other transcript-analyzing programs are sure to surface, each adding a new dimension to the diagnostic process. While having to input the transcript will be a deterrant to clinicians who work under time constraints, the analysis time saved, the amount of information generated, and the reduced amount of time required for organizing data will make the concept of language analysis more attractive in the diagnostic scene.

NEEDS FOR LANGUAGE TESTS

Where's the Rest?

Unfortunately, with the exception of some aphasia treatment programs that have pre/post test components (Katz & Nagy, 1982, 1983; Katz, 1984; Mills & Thomas, 1981), the above constitutes the list of assessment devices for language. The list of things that can be done with computers to improve the efficiency of the field is virtually unlimited. A look at the different elements of language diagnosis can provide some insight into what needs to be done.

Collection of Data

Computer-based receptive language tests will soon abound in the field of communication disorders. It is a bit surprising that someone has not already put together a vocabulary test that is the computer equivalent of the Peabody Picture Vocabulary Test (Dunn & Dunn, 1981). Technologically it is a time-consuming, but not complex task. And the advantages would be enormous.

Consider first the advantage of not having to manipulate the plates of pictures and record responses. The computerized version would present the pictures on the screen. When response is entered, the screen would present the next picture. Second, the computer would maintain counters to find the ceiling and basal levels for a test; stopping to count errors would not be required. Next, the computer would automatically score the results, thereby eliminating the mistakes made in that area.

The computer can calculate chronological age, find the percentile, stanine, and standard score and generate a report of the results in much less time than a clinician. And the report would more likely be accurate. Utilizing the computer, analysis can be more detailed because the computer can be programmed to sort, classify, make arithmetic calculations, and compare data. The speed with which it does these things makes it practical to routinely conduct deeper analyses than most clinicians now have time to do. Analysis of errors can reflect in-word-class versus out-of-word-class errors, errors of words with similar phonetic content, near misses versus gross errors, etc.

Computerization of tests such as the Test of Auditory Comprehension of Language (TACL) (Carrow, 1973) will reduce the amount of time spent totalling the various subtests. And the analysis of the subtests is what makes the TACL such a valuable test diagnostically. Another feature of computer presentation is the potential for movement. Animation gives the computer a significant advantage over still pictures in the evaluation of many concepts.

Using the computer to collect data for evaluation of expressive language presents more of a challenge. At the present time it is difficult to envision a computer that will take input directly from the client via microphone and translate it to something meaningful on paper. Technology at the present time is developing the capability of computer recognition of speech. However, even the best speech analyzers today have a word recognition list of only a few hundred words. Most are based on "teaching the machine the word." Teaching the machine consists of repeating the word into a microphone while the program averages the wave input to develop a model. That model of the word is compared against incoming information until a match is achieved. In this manner, the speech recognition devices are programmed to recognize specific speech input. This, of course, would limit the use of the machine with a variety of different speakers.

This is a long way from a device that can accept input from different speakers with a wide variety of speaker characteristics and can organize it meaningfully. The potential for such is there, however, and there is no doubt that eventually the computer will accept spoken input from any source and transcribe it into written text. That will truly constitute a breakthrough for language clinicians.

Analysis of Data

As was the case in articulation, analysis of data in language is probably the area in which the most progress has been made. One need only study the output of the *Lingquest Linguistic Analysis* and *Systematic Analysis of Language Test* (see Appendix C) to appreciate the depth of analysis that can be achieved with minimal effort and time on the part of the user through utilization of the computer. The author expects to see considerably more of these types of programs, with special analysis for certain disorder areas a growing feature. However, there is a uniform reaction to the print-out of results, which is "what do I do with all these data?" The author suggests that the greatest need presently is for analysis protocols that reduce the data to its most significant elements and that can provide the user with the specific information desired. (Sometimes less is better.)

Formulating Diagnosis

The comments made in the section on articulation apply here. Language will be more of a programming challenge, given the fact that language is affected by such a wide range of variables. Language diagnosis will require entering information on many other client characteristics such as intelligence, physical being, socioeconomic status, and any other factor which can affect the functioning of the individual as a whole. The complexity of language with all the underlying prerequisites will continue to challenge the field.

Prescribing Treatment

As with the articulation assessment software, the present language assessment software does not specifically address the task of writing treatment plans. However, the thorough analysis that is available when the assessment is complete makes the direction of treatment evident. Still, it will be one more step saved for the clinician when the treatment plan is an integral part of the diagnostic process.

Validating Diagnosis

Validating language diagnosis will again be achieved by verifying success of the selected treatment strategy through comparison of treatment results to standardized models. The validation process will be even more important for language, because it is a more complex behavior.

VOICE

Little has been done in the area of developing computer-based assessment material for voice. There is one computer-managed voice program for treatment that has some built-in assessment features for evaluating progress (Johnson & Child, 1984). This program (*Vocal Abuse Reduction Program*, VARP) will be discussed more thoroughly in the following chapter on treatment.

Perhaps the most promising avenue of computer-managed voice assessment can be found in the current adaptation of Visi-Pitch (1984) to the computer. The Visi-Pitch equipment has been used clinically to provide an easily read display of fundamental vocal frequency. In that regard it could be considered a feedback device. However, now it can be interfaced to an Apple II computer. This will allow for digital storage of the voice sample. The voice sample taken during the diagnostic evaluation can be analyzed for characteristics such as pitch, voice onset time, intensity, wave irregularity, and timing. Printouts of the information are available.

An interface such as this will provide the means of comparing fundamental vocal frequency characteristics of speakers with various types of voice dysfunction. Statistical models can be constructed of the various voice pathologies. This will permit the user to submit to the computer a sample from a client being seen for evaluation. The computer could compare the sample against the models and describe it in terms of statistical probability of wave fit.

In addition to Visi-Pitch data being submitted for computer analysi, data obtained through the Laryngograph (1984) can also be used. The Laryngograph analyzes input from two transducers held to either side of the thyroid cartilage of the larynx. The resistance between the two electrodes is directly related to the tissue density, which translates into how open or closed the vocal folds are at the time. Through simultaneous analysis of the Visi-Pitch and Laryngograph, models of the relationship between acoustic characteristics and physiological correlates can be constructed for various vocal conditions.

The noninvasive nature of the above means of study of the voice should lead to greater numbers of studies concerning various pathologies and define the characteristics of the pathologies in specific, quantifiable terms.

FLUENCY

One of the most promising computer applications to the quantification of fluency is in the area of measurement of voice onset time. Microcomputer-based strategies for measuring voice onset time have been reported

(Guillemin & Nguyen, 1984). However, the studies thus far on voice onset time (McFarlane & Shipley, 1981; Healey & Gutkin, 1984) have not employed the computer. As with the other disorders, computer-based measurement techniques are still in the development stage.

The potential is there, however. The disruption of air flow in dysfluent individuals has obvious and definable acoustic patterns. Hesitations, prolongations, and repetitions are definable acoustically in terms of voice-on versus voice-off times, phrasing, and syllabic configuration.

Simple voice-activated relays can be used to provide input to the computer which will permit the development of models of dysfluent behavior in terms of these characteristics. Computers have the capability of taking a simple on–off input and recording time ratios in milliseconds. Computers can also compare a sample of a client's reading of a known passage for voice-on, voice-off patterns and compare it to models stored in the computer. Again, this can provide the basis for quantifiable measures of dysfluency.

Repetitions can be detected by redundancy of syllabic patterns. Again, the field is years away from developing the models needed for meaningful analysis. But the technology is there; the challenge to the field is to apply what is already available in an intelligent fashion. Professionals must realize that technology will not stop progressing and the delay time between the emergence of new technology and applications of that technology to the field will continue to challenge our best efforts.

SEVERELY IMPAIRED

Probably nowhere has the impact of the computer been felt more strongly than in the area of treatment for the severely impaired, especially the neurologically and physically handicapped. Individuals with normal intelligence, but limited physical control, often are relegated to very passive roles in society, with little opportunity for two-way communication. The computer, and development of the low-cost speech-synthesizing hardware, have changed that dramatically.

Speech synthesizers can be programmed to "say" an infinite number of words. To obtain maximum intelligibility, models of words and phrases have to be refined by applying different production parameters. The refined versions can then be stored for recall on command. Thus the user can build a dictionary of words, phrases, and sentences that can be "spoken" by the computer on command.

In order for the user to output a spoken word, phrase, or sentence, the computer has to be signalled as to which phrase to use. The primary mode chosen for accomplishing this task is based on the concept of the language board, a board on which is placed a matrix of pictures (or printed words) that contain communication messages which the user might need. The manual language board required that the impaired user point to the picture (or word) which he wished to communicate. If the severely impaired individual cannot point with a hand, head pointers or other devices are used.

Digital processing improved the scheme. Pictures or words could be displayed on a monitor and a cursor moved from one picture or word to the next. The cursor moves from left to right on the monitor and at the press of a button begins moving down. A second press of the button causes it to stop on a particular block. A third press signals the computer to "say" the word, phrase, or sentence contained in that block.

The movement of the cursor can be controlled by means of a single switch. By simply wiring a switch into the joystick port, the computer can be made to respond to a single movement. The switch can be a traditional push button, a lever, or special switches that can be operated by the foot, head, mouth, or eyebrow. Thus a severely impaired person need have only limited movement of some part of the body to be able to utilize the computer.

To make the most efficient use of blocks, one word or picture might stand for a complete sentence. For example, stopping on a picture that depicted a blank television screen might be the signal for the computer to say the complete sentence "please turn the television set on." Thus the severely impaired were given a mode for communicating with the general population.

Bliss symbols (Bliss, 1965), which gained popularity as a compromise between Rebus reading and the printed word, have been adapted to the computer. Through the use of high-resolution graphics, the symbols can be printed on the monitor of a conventional microcomputer with ease. Software to create and utilize Bliss symbols on the Apple II microcomputer is now available (*Blissapple,* 1983; *Blissymbolics,* 1982).

The major applications for the severely impaired have been in the area of treatment and they will be discussed in more detail in the next chapter. In an effort to establish a formal tool for evaluating special needs of the severely impaired, Rushakoff and Hansen (1982) developed a program for assessing the efficacy of different types of single switches and determining the most advantageous switch placement. Data were in terms of mean normal response time.

SCREENING TESTING

The author has found the area of screening testing to be one that is adaptable to computer management. In an initial effort to study the feasibility of adapting an existing test to computerization, he chose to use the Fluharty test (1974). The study was completed in a Head Start program and the results were encouraging (Fitch, Davis, Evans, & Sellers, 1984).

The study compared the results of the computer-adapted version of the Fluharty test administered by trained graduate students to the results of the same test administered by Head Start center personnel. The Head Start personnel were teachers and aides whose education varied from high school to 2 years of college. None of the Head Start personnel had special training in communication disorders. The study found agreement of approximately 90% for the expressive and receptive language portions of the screening test. The articulation portion had less than 60% agreement. An analysis of the articulation portion indicated that of 50 subjects in the study, the center personnel failed 12 (24%) and the graduate students failed only one (2%). The indication was that the center personnel were too strict in judgment and the graduate students were not strict enough. Personal interviews with the participants in the study suggested that the graduate students made allowances for dialectal difference (did not count dialect differences as wrong) while the Head Start personnel did count them as wrong. This is the opposite of what might have been anticipated.

A second study using a screening test designed for the computer yielded slightly better results. The Computer-Managed Screening Test (Fitch, 1985b) was administered by trained Head Start personnel to 50 children (Holmes, 1983). Graduate students in their last quarter of graduate training administered diagnostic tests to classify children in the Head Start programs as "within normal limits" or "not within normal limits" (above minus one standard deviation on a standardized test). The results were compared to the results of the screening test administered by Head Start personnel to determine true and false, negatives and positives. Expressive and receptive language were again approximately 90% in agreement, while articulation was about 70%. Although the argument could be made that the lack of agreement suggests that the center personnel did not make judgments consistent with the graduate students, it is the opinion of the researcher that reliability of judgments for articulation generally is not as good as for language. When testing a child for language, an item such as "give me one block" will be scored more reliably than an item for an articulation test (a judgment on whether or not a child's production of a sound was within normal limits).

The Computer-Managed Screening Test has been administered to over 4000 children in more than 20 Head Start centers. Persons involved in providing services to those centers have reported to the author that the screening test, along with teacher referrals, is a satisfactory means of identifying children with communication disorders (Fitch, 1985b). The test also contains items for the examiner to mark for fluency and voice checks.

Results indicate that Head Start personnel overrefer on the screening test for voice and fluency by a factor of 5–10 to one for each child who actually has a problem. This is satisfactory, however, because professional personnel rescreen these children before administering a full diagnostic evaluation. Thus, center personnel screening for voice and fluency still save the clinician substantial time.

SUMMARY

The field is just beginning to realize the potential for using the computer in the diagnostic process. Most of the present efforts (and probably most of the ones to come in the next 5–10 years) are adaptations of established material to the computer. Eventually, however, rather than diagnostic tests being shaped by existing materials, diagnostic tests will be shaped to utilize the computer to the fullest. When this occurs, the field will experience a major advance in effectiveness and professionalism.

References

Blache, S. (1984). *BLACHE Phonemic Inventory*. San Diego: College-Hill Press.
Bliss, C. (1965). *Semantography*. Sydney, Australia: Semantography Publications.
Blissapple. (1983). Madison, WI: Trace Research and Development Center for the Severely Communicatively Handicapped.
Blissymbolics. (1982). St. Paul, MN: Minnesota Educational Computing Consortium.
Carrow, E. (1973). *Test of auditory comprehension of language*. Austin, TX: Urban Research Group.
Carrow, E. (1974). *Carrow elicited language inventory*. Austin, TX: Learning Concepts.
Chomsky, N., & Halle, M. (1968). *The sound pattern of English*. New York: Harper & Row.
Compton, A., & Hutton, J. (1978). *Compton–Hutton phonological assessment*. Hayward, CA: Carousel House.
Cooper, R., & Nielson, H. (1984). *Computer-aided speech production and training (CASPT)*. Salt Lake City: R.J. Cooper & Associates.
Dunn, L., & Dunn, L. (1981). *Peabody picture vocabulary test—revised*. Circle Pines, MN: American Guidance Service.
Faircloth, M., & Faircloth, S. (1970). An analysis of the articulation behavior of a speech defective child. *Journal of Speech and Hearing Disorders, 35*, 51–61.
Fitch, J. (1985a). *Computer managed articulation diagnosis*. Tucson, AZ: Communication Skill Builders.
Fitch, J. (1985b). *Computer managed screening test*. Tucson, AZ: Communication Skill Builders.
Fitch, J., Davis, D., Evans, W., & Sellers, D. (1984). Computer managed screening for communication disorders. *Language, Speech and Hearing Services in Schools, 15*, 66–69.
Fluharty, N. (1974). The design and standardization of a speech and language screening test for use with preschool children. *Journal of Speech and Hearing Disorders, 39*, 75–88.

Fudala, J. (1970). *Arizona articulation proficiency scale.* Los Angeles: Western Psychological Services.

Goldman, R., & Fristoe, M. (1972). *Goldman–Fristoe test of articulation.* Circle Pines, MN: American Guidance Service.

Guillemin, B., & Nguyen, D. (1984). Microprocessor-based speech processing system. *Journal of Speech and Hearing Research,* **27,** 311–317.

Healey, E., & Gutkin, B. (1984). Analysis of stutterers' voice onset times and fundamental frequency contours during fluency. *Journal of Speech and Hearing Research,* **27,** 219–225.

Holmes, E. (1983). *A computer-managed screening test of communication disorders for preschool children.* Unpublished M.A. thesis, University of South Alabama, Mobile.

Johnson, T., & Child, D. (1984). *Vocal abuse reduction program (VARP).* San Diego, CA: College-Hill Press.

Katz, R. (1984). Using microcomputers in the diagnosis and treatment of chronic aphasic adults. *Seminars in Speech and Language,* **5,** 11–22.

Katz, R., & Nagy, V. (1982). A computerized treatment system for chronic aphasic patients. In R. Brookshire (Ed.), *Clinical aphasiology: Conference proceedings* (pp. 153–160). Minneapolis: BRK Publishers.

Katz, R., & Nagy, V. (1983). A computerized approach for improving word recognition in chronic aphasic patients. In R. Brookshire (Ed.), *Clinical aphasiology: Conference proceedings* (pp. 65–72). Minneapolis: BRK Publishers.

Laryngograph. (1984). Pine Brook, NJ: Kay Elemetrics Corp.

Lee, L. (1971). *Northwestern syntax screening test.* Evanston, IL: Northwestern University Press.

McDonald, E. (1964). *Articulation testing and treatment: A sensory motor approach.* Pittsburgh: Stanwix House.

McFarlane, S., & Shipley, K. (1981). Latency of vocalization onset for stutterers and non-stutterers under conditions of auditory and visual cueing. *Journal of Speech and Hearing Disorders,* **46,** 307–312.

Miller, J., & Chapman, R. (1982). *Systematic analysis of language transcripts (SALT).* Unpublished manuscript, University of Wisconsin.

Mills, R., & Thomas, R. (1981). Microcomputerized language therapy for the aphasic patient. In *Proceedings of the Johns Hopkins first national search for applications of personal computing to aid the handicapped* (pp. 45–46). Los Angeles: IEEE Computer Society Press.

Mordecai, D., Palin, M., & Palmer, C. (1982). *Lingquest 1: Language sample analysis.* Napa, CA: Lingquest Software.

Palin, M., & Mordecai, D. (1982). *Lingquest 2: Phonological analysis.* Napa, CA: Lingquest Software.

Pendergast, K., Dickey, S., Selmar, J., & Soder, A. (1969). Photo Articulation Test. Danville, IL: Interstate Publishers.

Pickett, J. (Ed.). (1968). Proceedings of the Conference on Speech Analyzing Aids for the Deaf. *American Annals of the Deaf,* **113,** 116–330.

Potter, R., Kopp, G., & Green, H. (1947). *Visible speech.* New York: Van Nostrand.

Rushakoff, G., & Hansen, K. (1982). *Single switch assessment microcomputer program.* Technical report, University of Florida, Gainesville.

Schiefelbusch, R. (1980). The role of science in speech–language pathology and audiology. *Asha* **22,** 906–908.

Schuldt, M. (1983). *A computerized diagnostic and treatment system.* Orem, UT: Harding and Harris, Inc.

Sommers, H. (1979). Using the computer to analyse articulation test data. *British Journal of Disorders of Communication*, **14**, 231–240.

Stetson, R. (1951). *Motor phonetics: A study of speech movements in action*. Amsterdam: North-Holland Publishing.

Taylor, P. (1984). *A computer managed diagnostic test of articulation*. Unpublished M.S. thesis, University of South Alabama, Mobile.

Telage, K. (1980). A computerized plane-manner distinctive feature program for articulation analyses. *Journal of Speech and Hearing Disorders*, **45**, 481–493.

Templin, M., & Darley, F. (1969). *The Templin–Darley tests of articulation*. Iowa City: University of Iowa.

Video Voice. (1984). Ann Arbor, MI: Micro Video.

Visi-Pitch. (1984). Pine Brook, NJ: Kay Elemetrics Corp.

Weiner, F. (1982). *Phonological Analysis and Treatment*. State College, PA: Parrot Software.

Yorkstron, K., Beukelman, D., & Traynor, C. (1984). *Computerized assessment of intelligibility of dysarthric speech*. Tigard, OR: C.C. Publications.

9

Speech–Language Pathology: Treatment

INTRODUCTION

As in the case of diagnosis, it is inappropriate to discuss computer applications for the treatment of communication disorders without first discussing the basic principles of treatment. To do meaningful things in treatment, computers have to be programmed to simulate a meaningful model. The following characteristics are aspects of the treatment program which the author feels are most critical to the success of treatment. In addition, they are all characteristics which can be programmed into computer-based models for treatment.

Motivation

Perhaps the most obvious need of the clinical setting is motivation. Patients must have a desire to change behavior and a belief that behavior can be changed. The most critical element in establishing motivation for treatment is to convince patients that they will succeed. And an efficient way to do that is to design treatment programs that ensure a high degree of success.

Mowrer (1970) has indicated that clients need high success levels to maintain motivation. In effect this means that the treatment program in which patients engage must be constructed to assure high success-to-failure ratios. The author feels that for most individuals reinforcement for 75–80% of attempted responses is sufficient to maintain motivation (Fitch, Knott, & DeSalle, 1972). Treatment programs should contain controls that ensure the minimum level of success of 75%.

Treatment Effectiveness

One of the primary considerations in choosing a treatment plan should be whether it has been shown to be effective, that is, achieved the desired results. While this may seem offensively evident, if one considers most of the treatment paradigms that are used today, few have really been demonstrated to be effective in controlled studies.

The primary reason that treatment paradigms are not thoroughly tested in controlled studies is that clinical research is difficult to control. In one particular instance, the author was attempting to validate a treatment program and after 2 years still did not have the required data. The reason for the difficulty in assessing the effectiveness of a treatment paradigm lies in the fact that in a clinical situation, the clinician does whatever is necessary to get results. To be limited to one particular system under controlled circumstances takes away the flexibility the clinician must have.

For example, if a study is being attempted, and one of the "subjects," who is also a client, is not succeeding as well as the clinician feels he should, the clinician has to make a choice whether to continue the unsuccessful treatment plan under study or change to another in order to meet the needs of the client. Since client needs are always utmost in importance, the clinician must make modifications when needed. This takes away the control that is necessary to complete valid studies.

The effectiveness of treatment methods are often judged on the basis of how long they have been around and how widespread they are. A treatment method probably has some validity if many people have used it in many places over many years. However, judging the effectiveness of a new treatment method cannot be made on that basis. If a new treatment program is to be accepted, there must be some tangible evidence that it will do what it says it claims to do.

Efficiency

Almost as important as effectiveness is efficiency. Efficiency refers to the amount of clinician time required to administer a treatment program, the amount of client time required until acceptable progress is achieved, and the ease with which the program is administered. Two programs can be equally effective but not equally efficient. If one requires 4 hours of clinician time and the other 2 hours, the one requiring less clinician time would be preferred because of efficiency. The author has found that many clinicians have no idea how many contact hours they spend with clients having different types of disorders to achieve dismissal criteria. This should be a required feature of any treatment program.

Another feature of efficiency is preparation time for treatment sessions and time necessary to complete treatment records and prepare progress reports. The time consumed in preparation for one client is time lost in providing treatment time for another.

Pace of Treatment

It is desirable that treatment move as quickly as possible toward the terminal goal. Much of our students' training today, however, does not reflect realistic expectations. For example, in many programs students are required to complete weekly lesson plans. Lesson plans may contain statements such as "the patient will produce the /f/ phoneme correctly in 80% of the attempts" or "the patient will produce the /f/ sound in 8 of 10 attempts in the postvocalic position." Statements such as these are appropriate steps in treatment, but they should not be projected on a time basis. Learning is uneven. One day the client may have very good progress and move ahead at a tremendous rate. On another day something may have happened to affect him adversely and the progress rate declines dramatically.

Treatment should be at a pace that is appropriate for the client at the time. To have a lesson plan based on a specific time frame is not recognizing the nature of learning curves. Rather, treatment should be based on how well the client is achieving stated goals. If the client is having a good day, several levels of progress may be achievable. On a bad day, the client may do well to achieve no more than the level of the progress achieved the day before. But on both days, the structure of treatment has to be such that the client remains motivated, as indicated. That means that whether or not the client is having a good day, the success rate should not be below the 75% mentioned previously.

Simplicity and Ease of Operation

There is a great deal to be said for treatment programs that are simple and straightforward and that focus on the task at hand while limiting non-treatment activity. Elaborate materials, games, and reinforcement protocols may sound like worthy features in a treatment program. But these features can become the controlling aspect of the treatment session; witness the treatment game that is so good that clients (and sometimes the clinician) become focused on the game, not the treatment. Furthermore, time is valuable and treatment programs that require more complex protocols may require extraordinary amounts of preparation time. The amount of time that can be reduced in this regard will increase the efficiency of the clinician.

EVALUATING TREATMENT SOFTWARE

In Chapter 3, guidelines for evaluating software were presented. As a computer user, the author feels that it is good that the field has seen fit to encourage such a device. But there are times when the author feels that the evaluation of software is just that—an evaluation of how good something is as "software"—when the real goal of the evaluation should be to determine how well the program accomplishes its clinical purpose.

Few treatment programs have documentation concerning how much treatment time is needed to achieve certain levels of progress. However, there should be some description of the field testing process used to validate the software and some discussion of field test results. A technical manual, or section in the software documentation, should provide this information.

Since most computer-based treatment programs have limited histories, it is important that clinicians field test the software on their own case loads. Legitimate software distributors will permit their customers a trial period with the software to determine its applicability to their own programs. During that field test the clinician should ask the following questions: Does the software do the job better? Does the software do the job more quickly? Does the software simplify the task? Does the software make treament more pleasant for the client and/or clinician? Is the cost of the software reasonable for what it does? The greater the number of affirmative answers to these questions, the more valuable the software. However, even if only one question can be answered "yes," the software may be worth acquiring. For example, a program that makes treatment more pleasant, even if it is not more efficient or effective, may be worth using.

ELEMENTS OF TREATMENT

Background

Most clinicians do not realize the complexity of the task of providing clinical services. The variables that are involved in the most routine of

clinical treatment programs, and the data that must be acquired and analyzed constantly to make intelligent choices in the clinical setting, are
many and complex. The author became more aware of the actual complexity of the clinical process when he participated in a study with the
Veteran's Administration Hospital in Birmingham, Alabama, at which
project REMATE (Remote Assisted Treatment) was being developed
(Vaughn, 1980). The project will be described in detail later in this chapter.
Basically, a computer was programmed to execute a lesson plan over the
telephone with a client.

The study in which he participated was the first long-distance application
of the project (Fitch & Cross, 1983). At that time there were no lessons
already programmed, so the clinician involved in the study had to give
the computer all the information needed to conduct the treatment program.
Table III is a list of the variables that had to be input to the computer.

It required approximately an hour of clinician time to program a minute
of treatment time. A 15-minute treatment session required 15 hours of
preparation for the computer, because the computer is a completely passive
instrument that has to be told exactly what to do in every conceivable
circumstance. The persons involved in the study spent considerable time
reflecting on the actual complexity of even the most simple treatment
paradigm. The task that a clinician faces in the treatment processes, with
all of the variables that must be considered, and the decisions that need
to be made, is much more complex than it may appear on the surface.

Eliciting the Response

In the treatment process there must be the equivalent of a discriminative
stimulus, or something which tells clients that if they respond correctly,
they will be reinforced. This is usually accomplished by the presence of
the clinician and the setting. Additionally, there must be stimuli to elicit
a response. The most common modes of stimulation are pictures, written
words and printed words.

Clients are usually asked to respond with a motor response such as
pointing, writing, or speaking. The method of elicitation and the stimuli
to be used to elicit responses (which can sometimes be several hundred
stimuli per session) must be determined before the treatment session.

Judging the Response

After the client responds, the clinician must judge whether he should
be reinforced or not. In some cases reinforcement is given only in the
event of a totally correct response. However, in many instances the response may be reinforced not because it is correct, but because it is more

Table III. List of Variables Used in the
Computer Program for Remote
Assisted Treatment

Stimulus phrase to present to subject
Time to wait for response (30 seconds maximum)
Phrase to present to subject if wait exceeded
Number of repeats if wait exceeded
Phrase to present to subject after repeats
Step to go to after repeats
Number of correct touch-tone response
Value(s) of correct response
Random or sequential response type
Phrase to present to subject if response correct
Step to go to if response correct
Phrase to present to subject if response incorrect
Number of repeats if response incorrect
Phrase to present to subject after repeats
Step to go to after repeats

correct than previous responses. The concept of progressive approximation, or shaping a behavior that is in error gradually toward the desired end, is the foundation of most treatment.

Feedback

Clients must have feedback from the clinician indicating whether or not the changes that they are making are approximating the target behavior. Feedback is closely related to motivation, as previously discussed. A high percentage of the feedback responses to the client must be positive to sustain the client's effort in treatment. For children (particularly children with histories in which there has been a lack of success, e.g., learning disordered children), there may be a need for 90% of the feedback to be positive (i.e., reinforcing) to maintain behavior. For normal, achieving adults, there may be a need only for feedback indicating whether they are more closely approximating the target behavior. In the case of achieving adults, motivation is internal.

Clinicians have to make repeated judgments—perhaps several hundred times per session—concerning the quality of the client's attempts and must maintain consistent standards throughout the session. In working with behaviors such as word recognition, the judgment may be clear-cut. However, in tasks such as shaping articulatory behaviors, the decisions are not as obvious.

If the clients need reinforcement, and most do, clinicians must determine the pattern of reinforcement. Selecting whether it will be one-to-one, fixed ratio, fixed interval, variable ratio, or variable interval pattern may be critical for achieving the maximum efficiency with which a new behavior will be learned and maintained. One-to-one reinforcement is normally most effective in initial stages and variable ratio is more effective in achieving generalization. Selection of type of reinforcement and pattern need to be determined prior to entry into the treatment session.

Feedback needs to be consistent and provided in a systematic manner. One of the developments associated with the computer that will encourage consistent, systematic feedback is voice recognition equipment. Basically, the different types of voice recognition equipment have a common protocol. They accept waveforms of model sound productions (made via microphone by normal speakers) and store them. The client's productions are then compared to the model to determine how closely the wave forms fit. Feedback in the form of games or graphic displays is provided (Cooper & Nielson, 1984; *Video Voice*, 1984).

Vowels are more amenable to programming than consonants because of their longer duration and more consistent acoustic spectrum. However, as technology and methods of analysis improve, it is likely that consonant specification will become a computer capability.

If Not on Target

Clinicians then have to deal with what to do if clients' responses are not on target. Things that need to be decided include number of repetitions before moving on to new material; type of feedback (if any) to give clients for off-target responses; type of learning aid (e.g., cueing, prompting, modeling); and response mode (e.g., multiple choice, closure. Feedback for incorrect responses is an important element in a treatment session. Most clinicians have had clients at one time or another who withdraw from the session when given any type of negative feedback, or who become discouraged when they feel that they are not achieving at a satisfactory level. The welfare of the client as a whole, particularly with regard to self-concept, is most important. If that is not respected, treatment has little chance of success.

Criteria for Changing Difficulty Levels

The amount of progress made in any given treatment session should be the maximum of which the patient is capable. Translated into the real-life clinic setting, this means that clients will have good days and bad days. On the good days, they can move quickly on to more difficult material. Criteria should be established to move clients on to more difficult material when they are experiencing a high rate of success. The success is important to bolster the ego so that clients will be positive when confronted with material of higher difficulty levels. However, if they spend too much time at an intermediate level, that intermediate behavior can be overlearned, thereby making it more difficult to move to the higher level. While rates of success should be high on intermediate steps, complete mastery of a behavior should not be promoted until clients have reached the terminal behavior.

As indicated earlier, success rates of 75–90% of attempted material should maintain motivation for most clients (Fitch et al, 1972; Mowrer, 1970). However, the clinician must recognize differences between clients and adjust the success rate of each to that which is needed to keep that client's motivation high. The reciprocal must also be considered. Clients who are not achieving at a particular step in the treatment program must be protected against burnout by failure. It does not take many "no" responses from a clinician to undermine a client's confidence.

The best indication of whether the feedback and reinforcement strategy being employed in a session is working is to observe the rate of response or latency of response of the client. When motivation is high, response rates are maintained at high levels. When motivation slips, the response rate falls accordingly.

Avoiding Complexity: Focusing on the Client

The author's father used to admonish him when he got carried away with a task with a paraphrase of the KISS adage, "keep it simple, son." The need for clinical procedures that are straightforward, require minimal materials preparation, and are easy to implement is especially acute in the practice of a busy clinic. The clinician who has 10–15 clinical treatment sessions per day does not have great amounts of time to spend in preparation.

The author suggests that clinicians should concentrate their attention on the client and the behaviors being taught. To maintain rapport, and to be aware of the client's changing needs during the treatment session, requires a clinician who is attuned to the client and the task.

However, there are many other variables in the treatment session that must be controlled. As has been indicated, for treatment to have a predictable outcome, it must have a systematic structure. Stimuli, method of presentation, rate of presentation, criteria level for individual attempts, criteria level for changing treatment difficulty level, maintaining records for accountability, latency of response, and other factors must be considered. One solution for reducing the complexity of the treatment session for the clinician is to program the computer to attend to the routine tasks, thereby allowing the clinician to attend to the most important variable, the client.

Computers can make the treatment session much more "human oriented" by reducing the amount of attention that clinicians must give to the mechanical parts of the treatment session and permitting them to focus on the client. Using computer-based treatment, clients get the best of both worlds. During the treatment session they have the full attention of the clinician while receiving a treatment program that is constantly analyzing and responding to the different variables that are critical for success.

VALIDATING SOFTWARE IN THE FIELD

In Chapter 3 when evaluation of software was discussed, most of that review process consisted of evaluating the software from the point of view of "is it good software as far as software goes" as opposed to "is it good software for obtaining clinical results." Regardless of the proficiency of the programmer, the user friendliness of the program, or the esthetics of the graphics, software for communication disorders is only "good" if it accomplishes the task for which it was designed. And determining software's value clinically is more difficult than determining its quality as computer software.

Having made several attempts at clinical validation of material, the author is aware of the difficulty of carrying out research paradigms in a clinical setting. Despite this difficulty, materials should be field-tested in real clinical settings and the results of their use reported in the documentation accompanying the software. This report will provide clinicians with some idea of the application of the materials, but it will remain the clinicians' task to determine the usefulness of the software to their own clinical settings. Clinicians should evaluate software based on the following parameters.

Efficiency

The questions to be asked are, does it require less of the clients' time, and does it require less of the clinician's time? A program that interacts directly with clients may require more hours of the clients' time, but may require less of the clinician's time. Other computer-based treatment programs may require that the clinician be with the clients throughout the entire session. These are more efficient than treatment that is not computer based, because they reduce the amount of the clinician's time required to attain the goals.

Other than time, the difficulty of the treatment process should be considered. Here the questions that should be asked are, did the program make learning easier for the patients and did the program require less work from the clinician?

Effectiveness

The question that should be asked regarding effectiveness is whether the computer-based program delivers the treatment better. "Better" can mean that the goals of therapy are attained more completely and/or consistently. For example, a program that results in a terminal behavior being obtained at a 95% level would be superior to one that results in a 75% level.

In addition, the quality of the learned behavior should be considered. For example, a program to promote word recognition that clients generalize to daily reading tasks would be preferred over one that did not generalize. Often the quality of a learned response can only be evaluated in view of how it is integrated into the "whole" of the individual using it.

Cost Effectiveness

In view of the economics of many agencies today, this may be the most critical one. And very often the evaluation of the cost effectiveness of a program goes hand-in-hand with evaluation of time effectiveness, since clinician time is the most costly aspect of the treatment process.

Another cost consideration relates to travel—whether client or clinician travel is involved. Treatment programs that can be administered to clients at home, or nearer home, than the closest clinic may be an important consideration in sparsely populated areas. This is particularly true for clients with health problems or impaired physical conditions. The personal computer in the home and the potential of the telephone as a medium in treatment can have significant impact.

The following sections will include discussions of software that has been developed over the past 10 years. The reader should keep in mind that the software packages described were developed to meet particular needs of a clinical situation. They were not developed for general use by the field. While many have since become commercially available, the populations for which they are appropriate should be studied carefully. Clinicians who are looking for programs that are "just right" for their settings may be disappointed at limited offerings.

ARTICULATION

Fitch and Terrio

In 1974 and 1975, Fitch and Terrio reported on computer-based services in papers to the American Speech–Language–Hearing Association's National Convention. The first was basically a concept paper which discussed the potential of the computer in treatment. The second described a single-subject study on a child with a functional /s/ misarticulation. A network of filters, attenuators, and voice-activated relays were configured to identify the correct production of the /s/ phoneme by the child. When a correct production was identified, a switch to the computer was closed.

The computer was programmed to control several aspects of the treatment plan. First, it presented stimuli for the child to say on the screen. The child read the stimuli and if a correct production of the phoneme occurred, the computer flashed a reinforcing message on the screen. Then the computer presented another stimulus and the session proceeded.

The computer was also programmed to keep track of responses. When a predetermined criterion for correct productions was met, the computer presented stimuli with a higher level of difficulty. A predetermined criterion was also set for incorrect productions. If that criterion was met, the computer presented less difficult stimuli.

The child in the pilot study completed the program (correct production in spontaneous speech) in 2 hours of treatment time (eight 15-minutes sessions). While the study was a single case, it demonstrated the potential for electronic data management in the clinical management of speech disorders. The cost of the equipment in that study exceeded $50,000 and the complexity of the instrumentation was such that the treatment could have only been completed in a relatively sophisticated clinical setting.

Rushakoff

Rushakoff (1982b) described the utilization of a microcomputer and /s/ meter for providing feedback to clients. The program provided feedback for the correct production of the /s/ phoneme in isolation and in the initial position of the word. The computer kept a record of the total number of attempts, total number correct, total number incorrect, and total number that were incorrect but close to the target.

Other computer–technology interfaces were developed in the 1960s and 1970s in the area of training for the deaf and hard of hearing (Pickett, 1968). They were field-tested with limited success, but each added to the sum of knowledge of technological instrumentation. Since the goals of those studies were somewhat different from studies of articulation treatment with normal hearing populations, they will not be discussed here.

Fitch

The author developed a computer-managed articulation treatment program which was used in conjunction with Head Start programs (Fitch, 1985a). The Head Start programs, faced with funding cutbacks, were searching for more cost-efficient ways to provide treatment. The treatment program developed by the author for this situation worked much in the same way as the treatment program in the study that he reported in 1975. Stimuli were presented on the screen, but because the children in Head Start are too young to read, adult personnel from the centers modeled the material for the children. These same persons (some teachers, some aides, and some supervisors) listened to the child's production of the sound and pressed a key to signal the computer that the sound was either correct or incorrect.

As in the previous study (Fitch & Terrio, 1975), reinforcement, criterion for advancement to more difficult material, criterion for returning to less difficult material, and criterion for terminating the session were programmed into the computer. The Head Start center adult personnel assisted in the drill and practice work by modeling the stimuli and judging the correctness of the children's productions.

Figure 20 gives examples of screens used in Computer-Managed Articulation Treatment (Fitch, 1985a). Figure 20A is the instruction screen. Screens in Fig. 20B–D are examples of what the individual administering treatment sees during the session.

A

INSTRUCTION SCREEN

SAY THE SOUND, WORD OR WORDS WHICH
APPEAR ON THE SCREEN.

HAVE THE PERSON RECEIVING TREATMENT
REPEAT WHAT YOU SAY.

IF HE/SHE SAYS THE /S/ SOUND CORRECTLY,
PRESS THE '1' KEY.

IF HE/SHE SAYS THE /S/ SOUND INCORRECT-
LY, THEN PRESS THE '2' KEY.

--WHEN YOU ARE READY, TYPE 'GO,' THEN
PRESS RETURN.

B

SOUND IN ISOLATION

THE PURPOSE OF THIS STEP IS TO MAKE
THE SOUND CORRECTLY BY ITSELF.

/S/

C

SOUND IN SENTENCES

THE PURPOSE OF THIS STEP IS TO MAKE
THE SOUND CORRECTLY IN SENTENCES.

THE SUNLIGHT WAS BRIGHT.

TED WAS SITTING DOWN.

MY AUNT MOVED TO TENNESSEE.

D

SOUND IN CONNECTED SPEECH

THE PURPOSE OF THIS STEP IS TO MAKE
THE SOUND CORRECTLY WHEN THE INDIVIDUAL
IS USING HIS OWN SPEECH.

HAVE HIM TALK ABOUT ANYTHING--
A TELEVISION SHOW, A PICTURE, ETC.

1 2 3 4 5 6 7 8 9 10
(RESPONSE RECORD)

Figure 20. Computer-managed articulation treatment. (A) Instruction screen; (B) sound in isolation; (C) sound in sentences; (D) sound in connected speech.

The computer kept a record of the total number of responses, total number correct, percentage correct, data of each treatment, and highest step achieved. This information was saved on a data diskette at the end of each session. Another program was written to recall the data and print it in a tabular form and in a graph. Figure 21 shows examples of printouts of the program.

Field testing has been extensive (the programs have now been run thousands of times on hundreds of children), but it is still difficult to assess the effectiveness of the programs with given populations due to lack of controlled conditions in the field sites. The study most closely allied to this form of treatment was conducted on the language treatment counterpart of this program. This will be discussed in detail later in this chapter. In essence, it demonstrated no difference in effectiveness of computer-managed treatment administered by trained graduate students and the same treatment administered by Head Start personnel.

Weiner

Weiner (1984) developed a treatment mode based on minimal pair contrasts. The program was designed for children who exhibit open syllable syndrome, that is, who leave off the postvocalic consonant.

Pictures of minimal pairs are shown on the screen. The clinician signals the computer whether or not the child put the sound at the end of the word. Feedback is provided by the movement of the pictures across the screen. Performance records can be kept on diskette.

Summary—Articulation

At the present time, computer-based articulation treatment is making inroads in the clinic. Computer-based treatment is involved in the clinic process to the extent that it can assume many of the routine chores of the clinician. It can store and present stimuli. It can perform arithmetic tasks on incoming data, e.g., make counts on total attempts, number correct, etc., present reinforcement, and make decisions based on programed AI concerning whether to advance to more difficult material, move to less difficult material, or terminate the session.

The data obtained in a treatment session can be stored and later the cumulative treatment file can be recalled for reporting. By doing the above, the computer in articulation treatment allows the clinician to focus on the client and leave the routine clinical chores to the computer.

What remains to be done in articulation is the inclusion of computer-presented stimuli (through speech synthesis) and use of the computer as

INDIVIDUAL TREATMENT

REPORT

COMPUTER MANAGED
ARTICULATION TREATMENT

PATIENT'S NAME: WILLIAMS, TAD L.   FILE NUMBER: 85001
DATE OF REPORT: 5/10/85   CLINICIAN: JLF   SOUND: S

DATES OF THERAPY	TOTAL RESPONSES	TOTAL CORRECT RESPONSES	PERCENT CORRECT	HIGHEST STEP ACHIEVED
4/2/85	90	51	56	1
4/4/85	110	71	64	3
4/9/85	106	71	66	2
4/11/85	156	119	76	4
4/16/85	105	85	80	6
4/18/85	135	108	80	8
4/23/85	146	117	80	7
4/25/85	165	147	89	12
4/30/85	130	119	91	12
5/2/85	70	70	100	12

SUMMARY OF THERAPY

FILE NUMBER: 85001
SOUND: S

```
         12                X   X   X
         11
         10
          9
HIGHEST   8            X
STEP      7              X
ACHIEVED  6           X
          5
          4        X
          3    X
          2      X
          1  X
         ----------------------------------------------------------------
          1  2  3  4  5  6  7  8  9 10 11 12 13 14 15 16 17 18 19 20

                        S E S S I O N S
```

Figure 21. Report of results of computer-managed articulation treatment.

a "trained ear" to determine the correctness of sound production. When this occurs, articulation treatment will consist of the clinician training the client on the use of the computer. The client and computer will interact for the drill and practice work with the clinician as overseer.

Language is the area of communication disorders in which the computer has been utilized the most. Receptive language is especially amenable to programming because the client response can be more structured, e.g., multiple choice, pointing. The assault on expressive language has been mainly through the utilization of synthetic speech with the severely impaired. Since the development of software has been by disorder, the following discussion is divided into language software for children, language software for adults, software for voice, fluency, and the severely impaired.

LANGUAGE TREATMENT FOR CHILDREN

Wilson and Fox

At this time very little exists in the area of language treatment for children. The first widely distributed programs were developed by Mary Wilson and Bernie Fox at the University of Vermont (Durkee, 1982). With an exceptional blend of graphics and speech synthesis, they developed software that followed the traditional drill and practice paradigm, with the client indicating the response to the computer. The computer provides reinforcement through colorful, animated characters.

First Words (Wilson & Fox, 1982a) was designed to teach common nouns. The computer presents pictures of common nouns and through speech synthesis says the word which is the name of one of the nouns. A line indicator then moves from one picture to the next until a switch is activated. The child chooses the match by activating the switch when the line indicator is at the correct picture. The switch can be a press of the space bar on the keyboard, or it can be activated through the joystick port. The simplicity of the arrangement makes it suitable for very low-level performing individuals and ones with limited motor control.

First Words also includes various levels of instruction. In the first level, the match is indicated pictorially and the flashing line cues the correct response. In an intermediate level, cueing is dropped but the rest retained. At the advanced level, only the spoken word and the picture choices are given prior to the response and feedback is provided after the response.

First Categories (Wilson & Fox, 1983a) works on the same principles, but the goal is to teach word categories such as animals, body parts, or foods. Two pictures are presented and the child chooses the one belonging to the category being trained. Each category on level one has 5 nouns, and higher levels have 10 nouns per category. Both text and voice can be used. and the software has a testing as well as treatment mode.

Also from Wilson and Fox comes *Micro-LADS* (Microcomputer Language Assessment and Development System; 1983b). The stimulus presentation and response modes are the same as for the previous software and both testing and treatment components are included. *Micro-LADS* is a multiple diskette program, with modules for the following categories: noun plurals and noun verb agreements; verb forms; prepositions; pronouns; negative; "wh" questions and passive and deictic expressions. The programs can be used in either (or both) the speech and the text mode, so the programs can be used either as reading or auditory comprehension programs.

All of the above software programs have built-in flexibility that is very useful in individualizing treatment. Scanning rates (rate of movement of the line indicator), text, speech, response time, input devices, and treatment criteria can all be modified from a menu that appears at the beginning of each lesson. This gives the clinician maximum control over the parameters of treatment. In addition, records of performance can be maintained on diskette and reports printed out in an attractive format.

Other treatment programs are, at the time of writing, in development from Laureate Learning, the company started by Wilson and Fox (Wilson & Fox, 1985a). Their programs have won awards in many different competitions and have set a model for the field.

Fitch

The author developed software entitled *Computer Managed Language Treatment* (1985b) as part of the overall service program that he developed for Head Start. The software was designed to teach the concepts of colors, numbers and prepositions and included a general language development component. This program was designed to be used by teachers and aides in Head Start centers, so it was tightly structured. The computer was programmed to give instructions on the monitor to the individual administering the treatment exercise. Three-dimensional objects were used because young children respond better to stimuli with maximal cues.

After the child responds, the individual administering the exercise signals the computer whether the response was correct. As with the articulation treatment program, the computer presents a reinforcer and chooses the next stimulus.Criterion for advancement to more difficult material and less difficult material, based on performance, is included. Session results can be stored on diskette and recalled in convenient table and graph formats (as indicated in the section on articulation). The software requires that the child respond in different response modes. Formats for response through pointing, yes–no responses, multiple choice, and sentence completion are required.

A study was conducted which compared the effectivenss of Computer-Managed Language Treatment administered by trained graduate clinicians and the same treatment administered by trained Head Start personnel (Evans, 1983). The results indicated that there were no significant differences in progress between children who received the treatment from trained Head Start personnel when compared to children who received the same treatment from graduate clinicians. It was also found that Head Start personnel elicited more responses per time unit than the graduate clinicians.

Comments from Head Start supervisors indicated approval of the programs. They suggested that one of the principal strengths of the program is that it trains the people at the center to deal with communication disorders. These people have daily contact with the children, their parents, and their teachers. Since they are aware of the treatment goals, they provide feedback to the children, and teach others how to provide feedback to the children, so that treatment is an ongoing process.

The author chose to use software that presented instructions to adults working with the children, rather than software which required the children to interact directly with the computer. This was based on the fact that normally functioning preschool children have short attention spans and are distractable. The computer alone is not enough to maintain their performance. Furthermore, while the computer can be programmed to function within a range, it cannot respond to conditions beyond its range. For example, it cannot give permission to go the the bathroom or take care of a child who becomes ill. Preschool children need to have someone present to maintain their attention on the task and respond to personal needs. Finally, from the human engineering perspective, adults from the agencies need to be aware of the goals for children and be involved in the treatment process if maximum generalization is going to be realized.

Summary—Child Language

There is a tremendous potential for development of materials in the area of child language treatment, but the present time the materials are limited in the number of concepts and types of teaching strategies that are available. Also, the materials described above are for the lower functioning and the younger child. Materials for the older child, with more complex processing tasks, need to be developed.

LANGUAGE TREATMENT FOR ADULTS

Language treatment programs for adults have developed more quickly than language treatment software for children because adults are more able to work independently than children. Adults do not usually need the constant monitoring that children do. They can work through minor problems themselves and they do not need the strength and consistency of reinforcement that children need.

In fact, the computer has been found to be a preferred means of treatment with adults in many instances. Adults report enjoying working with the computer because it permits them to be in control of the treatment session. In addition, it eliminates the embarrassment of making a mistake in the presence of another adult. The machine feedback for wrong responses is seen as less judgmental than clinician feedback. And clients report that the computer gives them a sense of achievement. Learning how to operate the computer can offset the feeling of inferiority imposed by being in a treatment program.

Mills and Thomas

Mills and Thomas (1981) began efforts to develop programs for aphasics in the early 1980s. Mills had been searching for technology to facilitate the drill and practice exercises which are an integral part of treatment of aphasic clients. The *Word Recognition* software they developed (Mills & Thomas, 1983) integrated digitized speech, graphics, and real-time clock peripherals to perform the tasks. This software has a test as well as treatment mode.

The programs work in the following manner. Words are "spoken" by the speech digitizer. Four pictures, numbered for identification, appear on the screen. The pictures are high-resolution line drawings that are easily recognized. The client interacts directly with the computer. The stimulus is repeated if the client's response to it is wrong. If the item is missed twice, a flashing line box appears around the correct frame to cue the client. If the client makes a correct response, a visual and auditory reinforcer is provided, and a line box flashes around the appropriate frame. Client data can be stored on diskette for retrieval and report generation at a later time.

Several options can be software programmed. Clients can be added or deleted. Speech rates, response rates, and use of keyboard or joystick for input of client response can be specified. The software has maximum flexibility which most clinicians who work with aphasics would appreciate.

William Beaumont Hospital

Smith (1984) produced a series of software entitled *Cognitive Rehabilitation* which provide exercises for language-impaired adults. The software, developed in conjunction with the William Beaumont Hospital in Royal Oak, Michigan, provides interactive client treatment plans. Several different activities are available, including categorization, sequencing, association, and memory. The programs have consistent formats so that a client trained on one can easily switch to another.

Stimuli are repeated and hints given when an incorrect response is made. The programs have much flexibility in that the clinician may specify parameters for the number of times to repeat a stimulus when an item is in error, and may specify when to insert cues and when to terminate. An authoring program is included which permits clinicians to create lessons of their own choosing, or to integrate lessons from the different disks on to one disk for a particular client. The computer can keep group and individual records on lessons completed. Results include the percentage correct and the frames missed.

Katz

One of the most prolific computer programmers in the area of aphasia has been Rich Katz. Several of his programs are public domain and he has made countless free copies for individuals in the profession.

One set of programs, called *CATS* (Computerized Aphasia Treatment System) (Katz & Nagy, 1982), was constructed to facilitate reading skills. The reading subtests include the following: matching identical letters, numbers, and words; identifying the function of objects (words); identifying associated words; identifying synonyms; identifying words that rhyme; understanding sentences; understanding paragraphs—immediate; understanding paragraphs from memory; identifying correct grammatical structures; and solving simple arithmetic problems. Treatment tasks which are included in the software include the following: functions: identify the function of objects; question words: identify the meaning of who, what, and so on, in context; hangman: identifying and spelling words; sentences: identifying correct grammatical structures; short stories: understanding short paragraphs; math drill: adding and subtracting numbers.

Clients are initially supervised in the use of the programs, but all but the most severely impaired soon learn to use them independently. The software includes feedback for correct and incorrect responses and allows for repeated efforts on missed items. Performance records can be stored and retrieved by the clinician for reporting. Katz has been careful to field-test the programs in controlled settings and has good documentation for the technical studies.

Basically, an analysis of the results of clinical application of these programs by Katz indicated the following. First, there were no great changes in reading abilities. This is to be expected in aphasic populations and is a reminder that the computer will not remove the limitations imposed by the disorder. Second, clients were found to be more active in the treatment process and projected that they felt a greater degree of self-confidence and autonomy in the treatment process. Overall, they reacted positively to the computer-based approach.

Katz and Nagy (1983) also reported using the computer in the simulation of a tachistoscope to improve word recognition time and accuracy. The software, *FLASH,* presented words on the screen for a period of .01 to .8 second. Words were flashed on the screen in 2-inch capital letters in the same manner as flash cards. Display time for the words increased when the client had difficulty with the task, and was reduced as the client improved. Results indicated that all clients in the program improved on the task. However, as in the previous study, overall reading skills were not significantly improved. The by-products of client involvement noted in the previous study were also found in this study.

A third program, *SPELLER,* was also reported by Katz and Nagy (1984). Pictures of words were presented on the screen and the Client typed the word. A hierarchy of six cues was presented if the client had difficulty with the task.

In a summary of their experiences, Katz and Nagy suggest that "Many steps in the development of treatment software closely parallel development of a treatment task." As was indicated at the beginning of this chapter, a good software program must first be a good treatment plan. Software must embody all of the aspects of good clinical procedures if it is to be effective.

Katz has also developed a series of software for reading skills for aphasics entitled *UNDERSTANDING QUESTIONS* (Katz, 1983b), *UNDERSTANDING SENTENCES* (Katz, 1983c), and *UNDERSTANDING STORIES* (Katz, 1983d). *UNDERSTANDING QUESTIONS* presents pairs of question words, such as who, what, and when, and the user selects the target question words. *UNDERSTANDING SENTENCES* teaches comprehension of SVO (subject–verb–object) sentences. The user's task is to choose the word that does not belong in the sentence. *UNDER-STANDING STORIES* develops ability to find information in short paragraphs. Clients select statements that reflect comprehension of the material. The statements may be presented at the same time that the paragraph is presented or they may be delayed until after the paragraph is complete. All of the programs are turnkey, use a mutiple choice format and single key response, and can store patient performance on disk. Reports are formatted for graphic display.

Two other utility programs have been developed by Katz. One is *PICAPAD* (Katz & Porch, 1983), a program which computes all values and percentiles of the Porch Index of Communicative Abilities (PICA) Porch, 1967). Scores are input from the keyboard for the analysis. Subtests can be ranked by difficulty, scores can be displayed for comparison or correction, and test performance can be saved on disk. The software is straightforward and easy to use and can provide a hard copy printout. The second utility program from Katz is *KEYBOARDER* (Katz, 1983a), a program which uses sound and high-resolution graphics to familiarize new users with the locations of the characters on the keyboard. It has been found to be particularly useful for hemiparetic and hemianopic users.

Weiner

Weiner (1983a, b, c) developed three related software programs for adult language disorders, entitled *Aphasia I, Aphasia II,* and *Aphasia III. Aphasia I* presents a printed word on the screen and then a list of more words. From the longer list, the client selects the words that has a whole-part relationship with the target word.

Asphasia II uses the same format, but the goal is to develop association skills through identification of opposites and similarities. The response format for *Aphasia I* and *Aphasia II* is to press the space bar to align the matching words and then signal the correct match by pressing the return key.

Aphasia III employs the tachistoscopic approach in flashing words on the screen for quick categorization. The client is instructed to press the space bar if the word flashing on the screen is from a given category. The on-screen time of the words can be controlled by the clinician. It is suggested that this program improves response times and curbs impulsive behavior.

Vaughn

Perhaps one of the most ambitious of programs was developed at the Brimingham Veteran's Administration Medical Center under the guidance of Gwenyth Vaughn (Vaughn, 1980). Dr. Vaughn pioneered the use of the telephone as a medium for treatment for individuals living in remote areas or for whom travel was inconvenient. In the first studies, clinicians interacted with clients over the telephone directly by voice, or through mediating devices that provided for printed word transmission.

The inclusion of the computer into the paradigm was a natural progression. The computer project, REMATE, utilizes a mainframe computer (PDP 11/44) communicating with LSI 11/23 microcomputers (designated the line controllers). The line controllers communicated with a telephone line interface that translated touch tones into digital code.

Clinicians design the program to be presented by the computer. The variables which the clinician had to program were noted earlier in the discussion of the study by Fitch and Cross (1983). The variables listed there in Table III provide good guidelines for clinicians to consider in planning any treatment program.

The REMATE programming format works as follows. The client has a regular notebook for lessons. Each page consists of a plate of two to six frames which contain stimuli, such as pictures or words. The computer gives the item over the telephone and the client presses the touch-tone telephone key number that corresponds to the position of one of the frames on the plate. The computer then compares the response with a key to determine if it was correct or not. Decisions to proceed to the next stimulus or repeat the current stimulus are made by the computer.

As indicated previously, the author participated in the first long-distance application of REMATE (Fitch & Cross, 1983). The subject for the study was a 54-year-old woman who had a left subdural hematoma. She was 6 years post trauma and exhibited moderately severe receptive aphasia, severe expressive aphasia, and severe apraxic speech. She was confined to a wheelchair and had the use of only one hand. The goals for treatment were improvement of auditory comprehension skills and development of communication skills for basic needs.

Her lessons consisted of 10 plates with four frames each containing pictures. One- to five-word phrases were presented by digitized speech. The items were progressively more difficult as the lesson progressed. Figure 22 is representative of the plates used. The control sessions consisted of having the clinician present the same material manually (but in a different order). Sequence was altered to balance the role played in treatment. No difference was found between the results of lessons presented by computer and those lessons presented by the clinician.

The study demonstrated that delivery of communication treatment via telecomputer is feasible. As an aside, it was noted that the client responded very positively to the project. She nodded, smiled, and maintained an attentive posture throughout the lessons, even when no clinician was

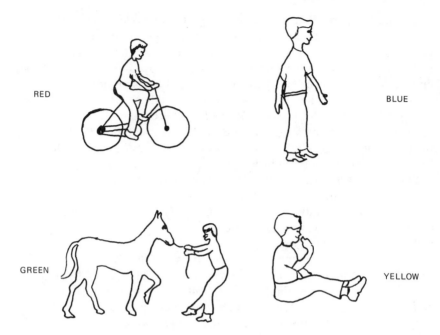

RED

BLUE

GREEN

YELLOW

Figure 22. REMATE study stimulus page.

present. This was not her normal manner, as clinicians in previous treatment periods found her to be passive and negative toward the clinical process.

Vaughn reports that a current study is under way in which the results of treatment for 50 clients are being analyzed. At the present time, the indications from that study are in agreement with the one cited above; that is, there is no significant difference between clinician-administered and computer-administered treatment (Vaughn, 1984, personal communication).

It should be noted that REMATE does not replace the clinician. In all cases, it is a supplemental treatment that is closely monitored by a clinician, and all of the clients have regularly scheduled face-to-face treatment with the clinician. It appears that *REMATE,* and other computer-based treatment programs, may have their greatest value in bringing quality treatment to persons in their home settings.

VOICE

As indicated in the chapter on diagnosis, little has been done in the area of developing computer-based treatment material for voice. One voice treatment program that is available is *Vocal Abuse Reduction Program* (VARP) (Johnson & Child, 1984). This is a program for use by clinicians and clients in the management of vocal dysfunction due to abuse. The program explains the physical properties of voice production through text and graphic displays of the physiological process. Additionally, it teaches patients how to use a wrist counter through which they can keep track of instances of vocal abuse. The data from the wrist counter is entered into the computer at each treatment session. The computer maintains an individual record for each client which includes data and text entry. Reports with graphs can be generated from the data.

As mentioned previously, one of the most promising areas of development for voice at the present time is in the computer interface of Visi-Pitch (1984) and the Laryngograph (1984). These are built so that they can output data to a microcomputer for analysis. The analysis can then provide a quantified basis for providing feedback concerning performance. Record-keeping procedures on performance can be maintained by the computer. Such variables as pitch and integrity of vocal fold movement can be identified and quantified by the combination of data acquisition equipment and microcomputer.

FLUENCY

Fluency, like voice, is an area in which much work needs to be done. Current technology provides the capability for detecting and measuring such variables as vocal onset time, duration, and syllable configuration. Once these measures have been established, they can be used to quantify performance. The quantification of performance will encourage the development of measurable goals. Immediate feedback can provide the means to more efficient establishment of fluency. Finally, the records that can be maintained concerning treatment performance will allow clinicians to examine the relative merits of different types of treatment protocols.

SEVERELY IMPAIRED

Nowhere has the impact of the computer been so evident as in developing compensatory language strategies for the severely impaired. The fact that the computer can be programmed to speak words at the touch of a switch offers a host of opportunities for the severely impaired. One of the first technological developments to recieve considerable attention for the severely involved as *Possum* (1982). *Possum* provided a means of attaining mobility for the severely impaired. The idea of using technology to help the severely impaired gain control of the environment was an attractive one and several projects were initiated. With the advent of the microcomputer, and its application as a logic device in environmental control systems, the cost of technology for the severely impaired decreased dramatically.

Wilson and Fox

Again, Wilson and Fox were among the first to use the computer with severely impaired patients (1982b). Their program, *Speak Up,* won several awards in competition for technology aids for the handicapped. The *Speak Up* software is a vehicle for the severely impaired person to obtain control over the spoken word. The "functional phrases" component works in the following manner.

Phrases and sentences which are functional for the client are stored in the computer so that at the command of the program, the computer will speak a whole series of words. Although a set of phrases was included in the software, the program permits the user to enter any phrase desired. Clients only need to press the space bar, or activate a switch, to use the program. The switch may be any type that can be used to complete a circuit in the joystick port. Even limited vocal output can be used to trigger the switch (Voice Entry Terminals, 1983). Key words from the phrases appear on the screen in two columns and an arrow moves from one word to the next. The speed with which the arrow moves could be programmed by the clinician.

The program works in the following manner. The client presses the switch the first time to stop the arrow in the general area of the target word. When the cursor stops, it begins reversing its direction slowly. This gives the client time to stop the arrow on the exact word with the second press. That press activates the speech synthesizer and causes the phrase to be output. Thus, two presses of a single switch can output any phrase in the computer.

The apparatus requires only the basic computer equipment, i.e., computer, disk drive, and monitor plus a low-cost speech synthesizer, thus making it a very affordable unit. An extention of the program was published later which permitted more rapid word retrieval (Wilson & Fox, 1985b).

Words +

Another unit which does much of the above, but with dedicated equipment, is *Words+* (*Words+,* 1984). The communication component of *Words+* uses the concept of the language board. The screen contains rows and columns of words, letters, or other stimuli. The client selects the stimuli to be output by the speech synthesizer by stopping the moving square block pointer on the target. The pointer first moves down until the client selects the row. Then it moves across the row until the client stops it on the target. Pointer control can be through any of many types of switches but, again, it requires only a single switch. The unit can output stored phrases, chain stored words together for output as phrases, or output words spelled by the client. Its stored vocabulary is over a thousand words and more words can be custom designed by the user.

Words + has the other modes which are advantageous to the user. It can be programmed to create simple drawings, present games for entertainment (many of which have educational or skill value), and control appliances (tasks such as turning lights off and on, or controlling the television set). The unit is reasonably priced, and several different types of switches are available.

Rushakoff *et al.*

In the early 1980s, Gary Rushakoff completed several projects involving microcomputers at the University of Florida. In addition to completing a dissertation in which he designed a course on microcomputers for professionals in communication disorders (Rushakoff, 1982a), he worked on several programs for the severely impaired (Rushakoff & Lombardino, 1983).

The *Florida Scanning Conversion Program* (Rushakoff, Steinberg, & Kreitzer, 1982) was a program to adapt existing software requiring keyboard input to a single switch scanning paradigm. The program originally required making changes in program commands so that the services of a programmer were needed. However, general programs are only useful to the severely impaired individual if they can control input to them. The scanning program provided a means of doing that for software that is open for modification.

Rushakoff, Condon, and Lee (1981) developed software for customizing a speech synthesized vocabulary for nonspeaking, severely physically handicapped individuals. The *Talk II* series consisted of four basic programs. The first, the *Talk II* program, includes three modes. The command mode is the primary mode for outputting chosen speech. The select mode provides a faster means of choosing words for individuals who can control it, by assigning keys on the keyboard for specific words or phrases. The sentence mode allows the user to store and retrieve sentences which have been especially designed for that individual.

The second program is *Word Editor,* which allows the user to put new words or phrases into the computer, or edit existing material. The third program, *Sound Editor,* does the same thing for the speech synthesis portion of the program. And the fourth program, *Update,* permits the user to remove old words to make space for new entries.

Schneier Communication Unit

The Schneier Communication Unit, Cerebral Palsy Center, Syracuse, New York, has been actively involved in developing software for severely impaired individuals. Several programs and strategies for interfacing computers and severely impaired persons have been tested there. Much of the credit for providing impetus for the work goes to the director, Carol Cohen.

Say It (Geiger, 1982a) is software controlled by a single switch. The program permits the user to choose spoken or written words and to chain them together in sentences. The vocabulary can be modified by individuals with no experience with computers. In this program, the client can access a dictionary of utterances that is categorized according to topic area. The utterance is spoken or printed through activation of the single switch.

Quick Talk (Geiger, 1983) is a communication program for individuals with limited ability to use the keyboard. The program is operated by the number keys and requires that the user be able to read. Using this program, the client can generate a personalized dictionary of words and sentences which can be printed or spoken and which can be modified if desired.

Magic Cymbals (Geiger, 1984) is based on the same concepts as above, but is designed for individuals who cannot read. Pictographic symbols are accessed again through single switch and output by speech synthesizer. It is appropriate for younger children or adults with severe involvement.

Tell-a-Story (Geiger, 1985) is an interactive program which tells a story to the client and then asks questions concerning the story. The questions are asked in spoken form and answers formatted as fill in the blank, true–false, or multiple choice. With the speech synthesized format, it can be used with nonspeaking physically handicapped individuals having visual impairments.

Sound Match (Geiger, 1982b), also from the Schneier materials, is a program which introduces clients to the computer by having them discriminate and match a variety of sounds. It is appropriate for children who are using the computer for the first time and who need instruction on listening skills.

Bliss Symbols

Clinicians who are familiar with Bliss Symbols (Bliss, 1965) will appreciate the *Blissapple* program (*Blissapple,* 1983). The program holds over 1400 Bliss symbols and custom vocabularies can be created. Using *Blissapple*, the message can be printed, spoken, and printed in Bliss symbols simultaneously. The program has many editing capabilities and can be used in conjunction with a printer with graphic capabilities.

A number of input routines are available, including scanning strategies, joystick selection, keyboard input, and special inputs through peripheral devices. The *Blissapple* program was developed in conjunction with the Trace Center, University of Wisconsin, and is available at a very reasonable cost. The source code of the program is also available so a programmer who wants to make modifications in the original program is free to do so. A similar program, *Blissymbolics,* is available through the Minnesota Educational Computing Consortium (*Blissymbolics,* 1982).

Summary—Severely Impaired

There are several other companies who are producing materials for the severely impaired. The variety of input strategies, dictionaries with editing capabilities, and types of speech synthesizers being used gives the user a fairly wide selection of devices from which to choose. Customizing a communication system for special handicapping conditions is becoming more affordable and can be highly individualized.

CONCLUSION

This chapter has presented a sampling of the types and varieties of treatment applications of computers. While it describes individual programs in some detail, The intent of the chapter is to provide readers with background that will help them in selecting from the many new products which will surely be available soon.

For the person interested in developing software as a career activity, this chapter should make it clear that the time and conditions for such activites are propitious. The application of the computer to clinical activities will have significant impact on the profession for many years to come.

References

Bliss, C. (1965). *Semantography*. Sydney, Australia: Semantography Publications.
Blissapple. (1983). Madison, WI: Trace Research and Development Center for the Severely Communicatively Handicapped.
Blissymbolics. (1982). St. Paul, MN: Minnesota Educational Computing Consortium.
Cooper, R., & Nielson, H. (1984). *Computer-aided speech production and training (CASPT)*. Salt Lake City: R.J. Cooper & Associates.

Durkee, D. (1982). Maple sugar and apples: A yummy way to learn. *Softalk*, 2, 170–172.

Evans, K. (1983). *A computerized program of language therapy for prepositions.* Unpublished M.A. thesis, University of South Alabama, Mobile.

Fitch, J. (1985a). *Computer managed articulation treatment.* Tucson, AZ: Communication Skill Builders.

Fitch, J. (1985b). *Computer managed language treatment.* Tucson, AZ: Communication Skill Builders.

Fitch, J., & Cross, S. (1983). Telecomputer treatment of aphasia. *Journal of Speech and Hearing Disorders,* 48, 335–336.

Fitch, J., Knott, M., & DeSalle, J. (1972). *Programmed articulation therapy (PRAT).* El Paso, Texas: Prat Enterprises.

Fitch, J., & Terrio, L. (1974). *Computer assisted programmed articulation therapy.* Paper presented to the American Speech and Hearing Association Annual Convention, Las Vegas.

Fitch, J., & Terrio, L. (1975). *Computer assisted therapy for communication disorders.* Paper presented to the American Speech and Hearing Association Annual Convention, Washington, DC.

Geiger, C. (1982a) *Say it.* Syracuse, NY: Schneier Communication Unit, Cerebral Palsy Center.

Geiger, C. (1982b). *Sound match.* Syracuse, NY: Schneier Communication Unit, Cerebral Palsy Center.

Geiger, C. (1983). *Quick talk.* Syracuse, NY: Schneier Communication Unit, Cerebral Palsy Center.

Geiger, C. (1984). *Magic Cymbals.* Syracuse, NY: Schneier Communication Unit, Cerebral Palsy Center.

Geiger, C. (1985). *Tell-a-Story.* Syracuse, NY: Schneier Communication Unit, Cerebral Palsy Center.

Johnson, T., & Child, D. (1984). *Vocal abuse reduction program (VARP).* San Diego, CA: College-Hill Press.

Katz, R. (1983a). *Keyboarder.* Los Angeles: Sunset Software.

Katz, R. (1983b). *Understanding questions.* Los Angeles: Sunset Software.

Katz, R. (1983c). *Understanding sentences.* Los Angeles: Sunset Software.

Katz, R. (1983d). *Understanding stories.* Los Angeles: Sunset Software.

Katz, R., & Nagy, V. (1982). A computerized treatment system for chronic aphasic patients. In R. Brookshire (Ed.), *Clinical aphasiology: Conference proceedings* (pp. 153–160). Minneapolis: BRK Publishers

Katz, R., & Nagy, V. (1983). A computerized approach for improving word recognition in chronic aphasic patients. In R. Brookshire (Ed.), *Clinical aphasiology: Conference proceedings* (pp. 65–72). Minneapolis: BRK Publishers.

Katz, R., & Nagy, V. (1984). An intelligent computer-based spelling test for chronic aphasic patients. In R. Brookshire (Ed.), *Clinical aphasiology: Conference proceedings* (pp. 159–165). Minneapolis: BRK Publishers.

Katz, R., & Porch, B. (1983). *Picapad.* Los Angeles: Sunset Software.

Larynogograph. (1984). Pine Brook, NJ: Kay Elemetrics Corp.

Mills, R., & Thomas, R. (1981). Microcomputerized language therapy for the aphasic patient. In *Proceedings of the John Hopkins first national search for applications of personal computing to aid the handicapped* (pp. 45–46). Los Angeles: IEEE Computer Society Press.

Mills, R., & Thomas, R. (1983). *Word recognition programs.* Ann Arbor, MI: Brain-Link Software.

Mowrer, D. (1970). Analysis of motivational techniques used in speech therapy. *Asha,* **12,** 491–493.

Pickett, J. (Ed.). (1968). Proceedings of the Conference on Speech Analyzing Aids for the Deaf. *American Annals of the Deaf,* **113,** 116–330.

Porch, B. (1967). *Porch index of communicative ability.* Palo Alto, CA: Consulting Psychologists Press.

Possum. (1982). Windsor, Berkshire, UK: Possum Controls Limited.

Rushakoff, G. (1982a). *Design and implementation of a course of instruction in clinical microcomputer applications for speech–language pathologists and audiologists.* Unpublished doctoral dissertation, University of Florida.

Rushakoff, G. (1982b). *The /s/ meter: A beginning for microcomputer assisted articulation therapy.* Paper presented to the American Speech–Language–Hearing Association Annual Convention, Los Angeles.

Rushakoff, G., Condon, J., & Lee, R. (1981). *Talk II.* Technical report, University of Florida, Gainesville.

Rushakoff, G., & Lombardino, L. (1983). Comprehensive microcomputer applications for non-vocal, severely physically handicapped children. *Teaching Exceptional Children,* **16,** 18–22.

Rushakoff, G., Steinberg, L., & Krietzer, J. (1982). *The Florida scanning conversion program.* Technical report, University of Florida, Gainesville.

Smith, J. (1984). *Cognitive rehabilitation.* Dimondale, MI: Hartley Courseware.

Vaughn, G. (1980). *REMATE: Communication outreach.* Annual report, Veteran's Administration Medical Center, Birmingham, Alabama.

Video Voice. (1984). Ann Arbor, MI: Micro Video.

Visi-Pitch. (1984). Pine Brook, NJ: Kay Elemetrics Corp.

Voice Entry Terminals (VET). (1983). Denton, TX: Scott Instruments.

Weiner, F. (1983a). *Aphasia I: Noun association.* State College, PA: Parrot Software.

Weiner, F. (1983b). *Aphasia II: Opposites and similarities.* State College, PA: Parrot Software.

Weiner, F. (1983c). *Aphasia III: Categories.* State College, PA: Parrot Software.

Weiner, F. (1984). *Minimal contrast therapy.* State College, PA: Parrot Software.

Wilson, M., & Fox, B. (1982a). *First words.* Burlington, VT: Laureate Learning Systems.

Wilson, M., & Fox, B. (1982b). *Speak up.* Burlington, VT: Laureate Learning Systems.

Wilson, M., & Fox, B. (1983a). *First categories.* Burlington, VT: Laureate Learning Systems.

Wilson, M., & Fox, B. (1983b). *Microcomputer language assessment and development system (Micro-LADS).* Burlington, VT: Laureate Learning Systems.

Wilson, M., & Fox, B. (1985a). *First verbs.* Burlington, VT: Laureate Learning Systems.

Wilson, M., & Fox, B. (1985b). *The fast access scan talker (FAST).* Burlington, VT: Laureate Learning Systems.

Words+ Portable Voice. (1984). Sunnyvale, CA: Words+, Inc.

10

Audiology: A Survey of the Literature

Audiology is a field based primarily on diagnostic procedures. Since the diagnostic procedures are established and quantifiable protocols, it would seem that audiology is a field that would naturally embrace computer technology. However, this has not been the case. Generally, audiologists have been slow to incorporate the computer into the routine testing regimen.

Interest in computer utilization was great enough by the early 1980s to motivate audiological equipment suppliers to begin including computer interfaces in their equipment. By 1985 some agencies began specifying that all audiological equipment purchases had to have the capability of being interfaced with computers (via RS232 serial interfaces).

The beginnings of clinical applications of the computer in audiology were somewhat different from early computer applications in speech–language pathology. The variety of applications was not as great and the number of individuals developing clinical protocols was more limited. However, those who completed the early studies in audiological applications tended to be more active in implementing follow-up studies, resulting in multiple publications by the small groups of developers.

THE COMPUTER AS A SIGNAL AVERAGER

One of the earliest applications of the computer was as a means of averaging evoked auditory potentials (Goldstein & Price, 1966). This was an insightful leap forward for the field and established the credibility of the computer as a complement to the audiologist. Many did not realize that they were using a computer because the instrument was often called a "signal averager," "evoked potential equipment," or "brain stem unit" rather than a computer with physiological data acquisition capability. In addition, most equipment for averaging signals was designed solely for that purpose so other applications of the computer component were not possible. This tended to draw attention away from the basic potential of the computer and it was years after this rather sophisticated use became established that routine types of clinical applications in audiology were attempted.

It is easy to overlook the quantum leap forward that was realized by the application of signal averaging to electrophysiological data management in audiology as indicated in the Goldstein and Price (1966) study. Clinically, it would be impossible to compute manually the voltages of the hundreds of points on hundreds of waves necessary for signal averaging. However, with the computer the averages can be calculated almost as quickly as the waves are being generated. Thus, a task that is impossibly difficult for humans became a routine clinical procedure with the utilization of the computer.

COMPUTERIZING ROUTINE TESTS

Wittich, Wood, and Mahaffey

In 1971, Wittich, Wood, and Mahaffey reported a study in which the computer was programmed to conduct tests for speech reception threshold (SRT) and speech discrimination (DS). In this study, the words for presentation were recorded on one track of a two-track audio tape. The second track contained a marking signal for tape movement control. A minicomputer with 4K of memory was interfaced with a masking generator and tape recorder through a peripheral interface module.

Stimuli were presented with an interstimulus interval of 7 seconds. When a stimulus was presented, the subject made a selection from a panel of five choices. The computer stored the sequence of stimuli so that it could detect correct and incorrect responses. If no selection was made in the 7 seconds, the response was counted as incorrect. SRTs were obtained using the 50% correct response criterion in a bracketing search procedure. Procedures for presentation of masking were included in the test paradigm.

A comparison of results of testing between the computer and experienced audiologists indicated that there were discrepancies in masking procedures, but that overall correlations of test results were significantly high. They concluded that "In general, the results of this study indicate that SRT and DS testing procedures are amenable to an automated treatment" (p. 343).

Sparks

Sparks (1972) tested the feasibility of computerized audiometry. The basis for his work was the growing need for large scale screening procedures.

> While it is imperative that institutions such as the military, public schools and industry be capable of performing precise audiometric evaluations of their personnel, the task is overwhelming when considered on a one-to-one basis between the audiologist and his patient. One way to meet the demand for accurate audiometry on a large scale basis is to employ the computer. (Sparks, 1972, p. 62)

Sparks found that correlations between manual and computerized audiometry were very high and no significant differences between the two were found. It should be noted, however, that only the logic for testing was programmed in his study. The tests were still administered by an examiner who read instructions on a screen and set parameters on the computer manually.

Wood, Wittich, and Mahaffey

Another study by Woods, Wittich, and Mahaffey (1973) was conducted to determine the feasibility of computerized puretone audiometric procedures. Both air and bone conduction testing were programmed with masking provided, if indicated. Descending threshold crossings using a bracketing technique with 5-dB intervals were employed to determine threshold. The computer was programmed to retest frequencies for which inconsistent responses were noted. They concluded that "Comparisons based on unmasked, air-conducted thresholds indicated a high degree of concordance between audiologist- and computer-determined thresholds" (p. 681). Masked, air-conducted thresholds and bone conduction thresholds were also found to have a high degee of consistency between the audiologist- and computer-determined techniques. In the discussion section the authors made an observation that bears restatement.

> The significance of the research presented in this article is not only that audiometric evaluative processes are amenable to computer programming, but also that procedures based on capabilities inherent in computer technology may provide a means of improving

the services currently provided to the hearing impaired by allowing the audiologist free time for direct patient contact, counseling and aural rehabilitation. (Wood *et al.*, 1973, p. 683)

Campbell

A study conducted in 1974 by Campbell confirmed the feasibility of computer audiometry. Campbell compared the results of audiologist- versus computer-determined thresholds for 36 patients at a Veternas Administration Medical Center. A unique aspect of this study was the fact that the stimuli were administered in a random-frequency, random-interval paradigm. This means 16 frequencies were being tested simultaneously in random order. To maintain the correct hearing test level for each frequency and set the equipment accordingly would be an impossible task for a human. However, the electronic manipulation of the procedure is easily accomplished by the computer.

Campbell summarized the findings by indicating ''Clearly, it is possible to use a minicomputer with a minimum of interfacing to perform basic audiometric testing'' (p.138). He also suggested that

The realistic use of the unique capabilities of a computer to develop audiometric procedures that complement the human limitations of the audiologist has greater implications for audiology than does duplicating the audiologst with a computer as a labor-saving device. (Campbell, 1974, p. 134)

Sakabe et al.

Computerized audiometric procedures have been in development in Japan (Sakabe, Ooki, Terai, Shinozaki, & Itami, 1975; Sakabe, Hirai, & Itami, 1978). In the first study cited, the authors describe a computer-based audiometric testing tool similar to the ones described earlier in this chapter. In the second, they describe the development of an audiometry data processing system designed to manage large amounts of information. Computerized audiometric procedures included air and bone conduction testing, Bekesy audiometry, and temporal tone decay. Also manually conducted SISI and DL tests could be input into the computer records. The main purpose was to develop a system which included the following features: (1) storage of large amounts of information; (2) sorting routines for identifying records with specific characteristics; (3) procedures for retrieval of information; (4) procedures for formatting reports of the data; and (5) editing capabilities;

The data processing system described by Sakabe *et al.* is, in essence, the format for maintenance of a large hearing conservation program.

Hearing conservation programs utilizing detailed systems of analysis will be discussed in Chapter 12.

BEYOND ROUTINE TESTING

Harris

In 1978, Harris discussed the potential for collection and management of audiometric data using the computer. In that article he states that "the first thing that should be said is that there is at present only the thinnest pretense of any standardization at all in audiometry even at its best." (pp. 1–2) He suggested that interexaminer differences in test procedures make the hearing evaluation more subjective than it should be. The lack of control of the temporal elements of the test situation (e.g., stimulus presentation time and interstimulus interval) also contributed to differences between examiners.

He also suggested that the accepted practice of using 5-dB steps in testing is too broad. If 5-dB steps are accepted in testing, and a one-step difference between examiners is permissible (±5 dB), it is, in effect, saying that a difference of up to 10 dB may be expected between two audiologists. Harris felt that this is not acceptable since 10 dB differences are said to be significant threshold shifts. His own studies indicated that thresholds could be consistently found to be within 2 dB. In the same article Harris (1978) stated the belief that the "yes/no" and finger movement method of responding leaves much to be desired. He felt that new testing paradigms can be developed using the computer which can more accurately assess hearing acuity.

Another potential in computer-based audiometry which Harris foresaw was the ability to program the computer to check its own calibration. There is the inherent potential to have the computer evaluate each tone generated and self-calibrate if the signal is found to be inaccurate. Compared to existing electronic calibration checks (performed once a month to once a year for most audiometers), the self-calibration capability of computerized audiometry is particularly appealing in that it eliminates the variance due to instruments not performing at specifications. He also noted that OSHA (Occupational Safety and Health Act) recommendations include acceptance of computer-based testing procedures.

In another article, Harris (1980) compared computerized audiometry by ANSI, Bekesy fixed-frequency, and modified ISO procedures for industrial applications. In a comparison of time efficiency, he found that the computerized Bekesy fixed-frequency testing procedure was the most efficient. ANSI suggested procedures required an average of 10.5 minutes per testee, ISO required 9.25 minutes, and Bekesy procedures only 3.35 minutes.

The Harris (1980) study was noteworthy because it was designed to compare the efficiency of different procedures, as opposed to previous studies which were designed to explore the feasibility of testing *per se*. He felt that the feasibility of testing had already been established, as noted in the following passage.

> Computerization has made possible a hitherto unknown standardization of stimulus presentation in tone duration, intertone intervals, and pattern of intensity levels; it has made possible a validation of each response of a subject in ways not available to the unaided manual audiometrist; and it has made available an instant and entirely objective calculation of HTL without depending upon the audiometric technician's memory, notes or clerical accuracy. Thus the judgments, and consequently the training, of the audiometric technician can be reduced to the barest minimum of initially instructing the subject and referring to the audiologist for individual attention those whom the computer labels "untestable." (Harris, 1980, p. 143)

This suggests that the audiologist will not be immediately involved in screening procedures or routine testing procedures on populations that are cooperative, such as adults in hearing conservation programs. Rather, his role will include working with populations that are suspected of having disorders or who are unable to respond consistently in a structured testing situation.

REVIEWS OF APPLICATIONS

The author has heard it said that when three articles have been published on a given clinical procedure, the field can assume that the procedure is one that will very likely become an established part of the clinical evaluation. Obviously there have been well beyond that number on computer applications—in fact there have been more than three literature reviews of applications.

An early review of computer applications was a chapter by Mahaffey entitled "The Measurement of Hearing by Computer" in a book entitled *Measurement Procedures in Speech, Language and Hearing* (Mahaffey, 1975). In Mahaffey's chapter there is a section entitled Clinical Applications. The section is two paragraphs in length and discusses two applications. While those applications were clinical in nature, they had not been replicated by persons other than the developers. Such was the state of the art in 1975.

In 1980, Levitt published an article entitled "Computer Applications in Audiology and Rehabilitation of the Hearing Impaired." The article reviewed much of the work discussed earlier in this chapter. In was evident in this review that the range of applications was small and largely still based in the laboratory. Levitt used much of the review to discuss potential uses, and stressed the power and efficiency of the computer in assisting the audiologist in adaptive testing. Adaptive testing refers to evaluation protocols which require an evaluation of each response of the examinee and choosing the next item to be given on the basis of the previous response. An example of adaptive testing would be a word discrimination test that presents more difficult material when the examinee makes correct responses and less difficult material when incorrect responses are occurring consistently. The above is a simple example. Percentages, consecutive correct-incorrect responses, response latency, and quality of response can also be included in adaptive testing.

However, adaptive testing by an examiner is only efficient if the response evaluation is a simple matter; e.g., was the response right or wrong. More complex response analyses, such as judgment of quality of response or degree of error, and adjustment of the stimulus presentation based on that evaluation, can quickly become too complex for human administration. The computer, however, can evaluate responses with multiple types of analysis and adjust stimulus presentation with no delay in the evaluation. This should encourage audiologists to develop testing procedures that consider multiple variables and adaptive testing procedures. While the premise is sound, little has been done in this regard to date.

The author reviewed the development of audiological procedures more recently (Fitch, 1983), noting in addition to the work discussed above the introduction of computer-managed hearing aid selection programs. In regard to widespread computer applications, he indicated, "Unfortunately, we cannot yet point to commercially available computer programs that enhance the capability of the practitioner who must test hearing and fit hearing aids on a daily basis. While much has been proposed, there is a paucity of computer-managed services for hearing testing, hearing aid selection, and rehabilitation." (Fitch, 1983, p. 32)

A more recent review by Stach and Jerger (1986) suggested that while computer applications continue to grow, there still exists limited innovative software. Stach and Jerger stated "Because microcomputers have quickly gained such popularity, there is a tendency to think that audiological applications of computers are equally novel. Actually, little of what is being done with microcomputers today is new" (p. 113). They noted that many of the computerized services had their beginnings in the 1950s.

They suggested that the current price reduction in computers has brought about a widespread move to computerize as much of the audiological evaluation as possible. Having been involved at their clinic with computers for years, they provided some insightful reflection on the danger of trying to do too much too quickly by computer:

> As we have begun to appreciate the immense power of this new technology and the extent to which it has increased our efficiency and productivity, we have also begun to understand the need to guard against the "technological imperative" approach to its application. That is, because use of microcomputers has profoundly increased efficiency and productivity, there is a tendency to want to automate those aspects of the laboratory and clinic that either can be done as easily without a computer or should not be done by a computer at all. Certain aspects of patient testing and data collection are enhanced by microcomputer use, while other aspects are much more appropriately carried out by the audiologist (Stach and Jerger, 1986, p. 113).

In addition to the types of applications noted above, they noted that measurement of the acoustic reflex has been demonstrated to be an effective clinical procedure. The use of the computer for signal averaging reduces the need for filtering for noise reduction and allows the analysis of undistorted temporal characteristics of the reflex. They indicate that this results in more definitive threshold detection. Computer utilization in reflex testing also reduces the amount of time required for the test and the analysis of the reflex is performed more quickly and thoroughly.

Stach and Jerger (1985) also reported using the microcomputer with cochlear implants. The multichannel implant requires adjustment of as many as 21 different electrodes. A map is created which contains the level of current necessary to reach threshold of audibility and maintain maximum comfort level. They report that the microcomputer is especially useful in keeping a record of the values contained in the implant map. It has also been used in the psychophysical evaluation of implant function.

The decision-making capability of the microcomputer, which in fact is a computational algorithm, is suggested by Stach and Jerger. They use the microcomputer to analyze latency and interval characteristics of ABR responses in order to classify them as normal, abnormal, or questionable. Comparison of use of the algorithm with a group of 34 clients with confirmed acoustic neuromas and 34 clients with cochlear hearing loss indicated that the algorithm was valid for differentiating cochlear and retrocochlear hearing loss.

REHABILITATION

Little has been done in using the computer in the rehabilitation process. The most notable efforts have been in the area of education of the deaf, which is beyond the scope of this book. For an idea of some applications in that area, the reader is directed to a list of suggested material at the end of the chapter. This will provide at least a starting point for the person interested in pursuing information on the computer in rehabilitation.

SUMMARY

The computerization of hearing testing has been demonstrated to be clinically feasible for a variety of testing procedures. However, only evoked potential signal averaging has become a professional standard for the field. Currently, the most widespread application of the microcomputer appears to be its use as a word processor for report preparation. The question of whether the microcomputer will become the centerpiece of the audiologist's equipment has yet to be answered. At the present time the literature reflects that the potential for extensive use of the microcomputer in the testing situation is feasible. In the next chapter the role of the microcomputer in the diagnostic and treatment processes will be discussed.

References

Campbell, R. (1974). Computer audiometry. *Journal of Speech and Hearing Research, 17,* 134–140.
Fitch, J. (1983). Computer based services for the hearing health professional. *Hearing Journal, 36,* 31–34.
Goldstein, R., & Price, L. (1966). Clinical use of EEA with an average response computer: A case report. *Journal of Speech and Hearing Disorders, 31,* 75–78.
Harris, J. (1978). Proem to a quantum leap in audiometric data collection and managment. *Journal of Auditory Research, 18,* 1–29.
Harris, J. (1980). A comparison of computerized audiometry by ANSI, Bekesy fixed-frequency, and modified ISO procedures in an industrial hearing conservation program. *Journal of Auditory Research, 20,* 143–167.
Levitt, H. (1980). Computer applications in audiology and rehabilitation of the hearing impaired. *Journal of Communication Disorders, 13,* 471–481.
Mahaffey, R. (1975). The measurement of hearing by computer. In S. Singh (Ed.), *Measurement procedures in speech, hearing and language* (pp. 323–341). Baltimore: University Park Press.
Sakabe, N., Hirai, Y., & Itami, E. (1978). Modification and application of the computerized automatic audiometer. *Scandinavian Audiologica 7,* 105–109.
Sakabe, N., Ooki, T., Terai, E., Shinozaki, K., & Itami, E. (1975). A computereized automatic audiometer. *Scandinavian Audiologica, 4,* 75–81.
Sparks, D. (1972). The feasibility of computerized audiometry. *Journal of Auditory Research, 12,* 62–66.
Stach, B., & Jerger, J. (1986). Microcomputer applications in audiology. In J. Northern (Ed.), *The personal computer for speech, language, and hearing professionals* (p. 113–134). Boston: Little, Brown & Co.

Wittich, W., Wood, T., & Mahaffey, R. (1971). Computerized speech audiometric procedures. *Journal of Auditory Research,* **11,** 335–344.

Wood, T., Wittich, W., & Mahaffey, R. (1973). Computerized pure-tone audiometric procedures. *Journal of Speech and Hearing Disorders,* **16,** 676–684.

Suggested Readings

Cook, G., & Creech, H. (1983). Reliability and validity of computer hearing tests. *Hearing Instrucments,* **34,** 10–13, 39.

Fritze, W. (1978). A computer-controlled binaural balance test. *Acta Otolaryngologica* **86,** 89–92.

Harris, D. (1979a). Microprocessor versus self-recording audiometer in industry. *Journal of Auditory Research,* **19,** 137–149.

Harris, D. (1979b). Microprocessor, self-recording and manual audiometry. *Journal of Auditory Research,* **19,** 159–166.

Kamm, C., Carterette, E., Morgan, D., & Dirks, D. (1980). Use of digitaized speech materials in audiological research. *Journal of Speech and Hearing Research,* **23,** 709–721.

Lehnhardt, E., Battmer, R., & Becker, D. (1980). Storage of audiometric data—online—with a small computer. *Archives of Otorhinolaryngology,* **226,** 199–206.

Levinson, S., & Liberman, M. (1981). Speech recognition by computer. *Scientific American,* **26,** 64–76.

Levitt, H., Slosberg, R., Hawie, D., & Mazer, R. 1978. Computer-based techniques for the enhancement of clinical techniques, *Asha,* **20,** 398–402.

Nickerson, R., Kalikow, D., & Stevens, K. (1976). Computer-aided speech training for the deaf. *Journal of Speech and Hearing Disorders,* **41,** 120–132.

11

Audiology: Diagnosis and Treatment

For a discussion of the use of the computer in audiology to be meaningful, the diagnostic and treatment processes themselves must have a definition that is common to the author and reader. It has been noted several times previously in this book that perhaps the most important feature of the computer is that it forces the user to approach tasks in a logical fashion. The use of the computer in audiology presupposes that audiological procedures are logical processes. The purpose of the first section of this chapter will be to discuss the logic involved in the clinical audiological diagnosis process.

Two of the general procedures involved in the diagnostic process are case management and individual test management. Case management refers to the selection, interpretation, and prescription aspects of the diagnostic process. Individual test management deals with the administration and scoring of specific tests in the audiological battery.

CASE MANAGEMENT

Elements of Case Management

The overall management of a client who is being seen for a hearing evaluation requires much more than simply the administration of a series of individual tests. Initially, it must be decided tests should be given, what information other than test data needs to be collected, and the sequence in which these things will be accomplished. Decisions of this nature are usually made by studying the case history of the client and obtaining further information in an initial intake interview.

As the battery of testing progresses, the audiologist is constantly making an evaluation of the client's responses and adapting to his needs. During individual tests the audiologist analyzes each response to determine if it is a valid one. Such factors as anxiety, fatigue, and lack of attention to task can negate response validity. The validity of each test as a whole must be assessed. The audiologist also studies the results of the test just completed to determine the next test to administer. The audiologist selects a sequence and order for tests which yield what he believes to be the most accurate results.

When the battery is completed, the audiologist analyzes the test results, considers them in view of information gained from the case history and interview, and formulates a diagnosis. The audiologist may administer additional tests, or refer the client for evaluation by other professionals to confirm or deny his findings using a differential diagnosis strategy.

When all of the above data have been collated into a meaningful compendium of information, the audiologist reports the findings of the evaluation. No matter how skillfully a hearing evaluation is conducted, it is only meaningful to the extent that the results can be understood by others. Thus the reporting process is a critical element. Reporting is usually done verbally and in writing, both of which require specific skills.

Most would agree that effective case management requires intelligence, training, and experience. The audiologist who approaches the task with a deficit in any one of those areas cannot be maximally effective.

The Computer in Case Management

At the present time the field cannot point to a computerized algorithm to do the functions mentioned above. In fact, there has been little done in the area of computerized case management. The author feels that the main reason this is true has to do with the relative immaturity of the computer as compared to an audiologist. This requires some explanation.

One of the most obvious shortcomings of the computer is its inability to interact with the client (Sparks, 1972). The effective audiologist does many things to facilitate the evaluation process. First, human visual cues such as smiling, eye contact, and body posture from the examiner can make examinees feel assured and motivated to perform at their best. The audiologist can draw upon previous experience to make decisions concerning what to say and do with a client. Campbell (1974) stated "The deficit of the computer that is more difficult to cope with is the extremely limited information available to it both before and during testing." (p. 139) Present-day computers do not have the capability of processing visual and auditory stimuli and comparing them to past experiences. While computers can be programmed to learn, the complexity of the learning process for human interaction is such that it cannot at this time be duplicated by artificial intelligence.

Second, computers have limited means of responding. Even the best speech synthesizer is easily identified as nonhuman and devoid of empathy. And there is no computer correlate for a smile or frown. Communication between the computer and client is limited in mode, content, and nuance. (Of course, this is not to say that all audiologists possess the total range of communication skills.)

In addition, "The computer does not have intuitive feelings about patients' attitudes toward the audiometric evaluation, as a clinician often has, and a clinician's intuition can sometimes play a decisive role in establishing reliable thresholds in difficult-to-test patients" (Sparks, 1972, p. 66). At present, computers respond only within prescribed ranges of choice and cannot respond to unique or novel input, other than to identify it as being unique or novel. The phrase "that does not compute" has been used for years and sums up the computer's response to anything outside its realm of information.

However, the same can be said for individuals learning to be audiologists. When something occurs that they have not seen before, it "does not compute" and its significance may be lost. Only after audiologists have had past experiences to which new experiences can be related can they be most effective. This suggests that the more experience audiologists gain, the more effective they will be in hearing testing.

This is where the concept of computer immaturity enters. Computers today are like children who have limited communication skills and limited life experiences. They can respond only in structured situations to limited information. Until computers have the capacity for communication that is of the level of sophistication of human communication, and until they can store experiences and integrate them in the fashion that the human brain does, they will be of little value in case management. Such a capability for computers is not in the foreseeable future.

There are, however, areas in which computer management could be, but has not been, applied. One such area is that of case history management. At the present time, the typical case history is taken by having the client complete a form with specific questions. The audiologist reads the case history and in an interview with the client asks questions based on the information contained therein. The computer could assist in the process by providing a means of obtaining a case history through "intelligent" interaction with the client. It could be done in the following manner.

There is often a section on the case history form with instructions similar to "Circle any of the following that you have experienced" followed by a list of symptoms such as "ringing in the ears," "dizziness," "nausea." The audiologist notes the items marked and follows up by asking more about the ones circled. The computer could do the same thing by presenting a menu with the questions, and following up each symptom indicated with a set of relevant questions, the answers to which would help to specify the disorder.

For example, in response to the client indicating dizziness, the computer could present a series of multiple-choice answers which would help to describe the symptom more fully. It could specify the temporal and spatial circumstances, i.e., when and where dizziness is experienced. It could ask questions that would help identify the possibility of vestibular involvement, i.e., questions about balance, and it probe into possible physical correlates, i.e., with questions related to circulatory distress, injuries to the head, etc. In addition, it could ask questions specific to a set of symptoms, e.g., questions related to key words such as "head injury" and "ringing in the ears."

The value that such a case history procedure could have is two-fold. First, having the follow-up questions asked before the client enters the evaluation would result in time savings. Second, such a case history procedure would be of value to less experienced audiologists and audiologists-in-training in that it would assure them that the correct follow-up questions had been asked. In addition to the above, the computer could be programmed to recommend tests to be given and the sequence in which they might be administered most effectively.

The above requires programming that is technologically feasible, but which requires the time and talents of audiologists who have the clinical experience and who know what questions should be asked. Again, the value of computerized management lies in the value of the information with which the computer is programmed.

A second potential area of case management by computer can be found in the quantification and standardization of analysis of test results. At present the experienced audiologist analyzes the test results and decides what additional tests to give and when to stop testing and produce a diagnosis. The computer can be programmed to accomplish the same task, and, if programmed with the information on which experienced audiologists make the decisions, it will make those same decisions.

The value of such an analysis would be that the computer considers all the possibilities each time and is not biased or impaired by conditions. Audiologists are subject to all the human weaknesses that distort judgment, i.e., not feeling well, fatigue, being rushed for time, or a million other reasons. While programming a computer with all the information and algorithms that are used by an experienced clinician would require a sizable investment of time and energy, once the program was written it could serve an unlimited number of persons in unlimited numbers of settings. And once a new piece of information or new algorithm important for hearing evaluation was identified, the program could be updated.

The only area in which serious inroads are being made in case management at the present time is in the area of reporting. The use of the computer for word processing capabilities in report preparation is becoming widespread. In addition, audiological equipment is now routinely becoming equipped with RS232 serial interface cards so that information can be transferred directly between the computer and the testing equipment.

This opens the possibility of programming the computer to act on the information being input in any number of ways, and to format time-saving reports of the results and analysis. The data can also be stored for future retrieval and analysis. The efficiency of the computer in this area will break ground for the inclusion of the previously listed areas of potential development for computer management.

INDIVIDUAL TEST MANAGEMENT

The use of the computer in the management of individual tests has received more attention. As indicated before, the computer has been programmed to administer pure tone threshold tests (Sparks, 1972; Wood, Wittich, & Mahaffey, 1973; Campbell, 1974; Sakabe, Hirai, & Itami, 1978; and Harris, 1980), speech reception threshold and word discrimination testing (Wittich, Wood, & Mahaffey, 1971), the Temporal Tone Decay test (Sakabe et al., 1978), Alternate Binaural Loudness Balance (ABLB) test (Fritze, 1978), and acoustic reflex (Jerger & Hayes, 1983; Stach & Jerger, 1984). While a great deal can be said for the efforts thus far, the only routine clinical evaluation in which the computer is presently utilized as an integral feature is in signal averaging for brain stem response (BSR) (Skinner, 1978). Since the technology exists, and the efficacy of such testing has been demonstrated, why has the computer not become the centerpiece of the audiology suite?

There are several reasons that the computer has not yet come of age in audiology. First, a review of the above studies will demonstrate that the hardware on which they were developed was either mainframe computers or minicomputers, in the price range of $25,000 +. Few clinical, research, or university programs could support that investment. In addition, the programs written for those computers could not be readily translated into software for the microcomputers. Microcomputers have only become widely available at low cost in the past few years, and the peripherals for microcomputers needed to support the programs above have only become available even more recently.

Another reason computerization of audiology has not occurred more rapidly has to do with the marketability of computers to audiologists in the field. In other words, even if computers were available, would they be used by audiologists? In 1981 the author had several informal discussions with representatives of major audiological equipment manufacturers concerning computers. When asked why they were not doing more to develop computers in audiology, they all gave slightly different responses, but the common thread through the explanations was that audiologists (who controlled the funds for purchasing equipment) were not ready for them. One representative put it succinctly in saying "they still want the knobs and dials. They're not ready to accept a keyboard." Audiologists whose only training was with conventional equipment could hardly be expected to embrace a technology which had yet to be subjected to the test of time. It was with a good deal of caution that they approached the computer initially.

Still another reason that the computer did not arrive in the audiology marketplace sooner deals with manufacturers of audiological equipment. Audiological equipment is not a high-volume business—it is known as a *thin* market. Mark-up of prices must be substantial to offset the expense of development and advertising, which is necessary to market the product. Manufacturers could hardly be expected to retool and begin producing completely different equipment without some delay, even if there had been a market for it.

What has transpired is a gradual shift from the traditional audiological equipment configuration to the inclusion of the microcomputer. Many audiometers have become equipped with RS232 ports, which are interface boards which allow them to send and accept signals from a microcomputer. It is expected that the shift will move more toward integrated systems centered around the microcomputer.

Eventually audiology will most likely go the route that the retail store, the supermarket, the airline reservation office, and the insurance office have gone—to computers as the main piece of data-processing equipment. In addition to the flexibility that the computer provides, the cost savings will be substantial. A digital-to-analog output board which can duplicate all of the signals of the most expensive computer can be purchased for less than $1000 today, and the price will probably continue to decrease. This board can be interfaced with a microcomputer (costing less than $1000) which can be programmed to conduct all of the tests now available plus allow infinite flexibility through creative programming by the user.

The last ingredient is software development and manufacturers who will produce special-purpose digital-to-analog boards. As of this writing, a board has just come on the market which can change a microcomputer into an audiometer. One has only to plug it into the expansion slot of the microcomputer, plug in the earphones, and load the software; all for an advertised cost of less than $600 (MAB-100, 1984).

While there appears to be great promise, it is suggested that the transition to computerized audiology will be a very gradual process for the most part. There are, however, areas of audiological management which have embraced computers with a fervor. Those will be the next topics of discussion.

HEARING AID SELECTION

It is perhaps only natural that hearing aid selection would be subjected to computer analysis, given the fact that there has been a long history of controversy surround the hearing aid fitting process without a great deal of success (Ross, 1978). The computer's ability to manipulate numbers, and the theoretical position that hearing aid gain contours can be fitted to hearing loss contours, suggest a logic to computer-analyzed fittings.

Hertzano, Levitt, and Slosberg

In 1979, Hertzano, Levitt, and Slosberg presented a paper that suggested the feasibility of using the computer to aid in hearing aid selection. They described a database that stored the physical characteristics of amplification (e.g., frequency response and harmonic distortion) which had been taken on a standard 2-cc coupler. The characteristics of the hearing aids stored in the database were compared to measurements on the same coupler for a master hearing aid. Commercial hearing aids that most closely approximate the optimum characteristics for a given client are identified by the analysis.

Craig and Seigenthaler

Craig and Seigenthaler (1981) described a system named Preliminary Hearing Aid Selection System (PHASS). Ten characteristics of hearing aids were selected for analysis. They included four acoustic features: full-on gain, reference test gain, SSPL-90 (SSPL: signal sound pressure level) measured according to the high frequency averaging, and frequency-gain characteristics. The six other descriptors included type of aid (e.g., behind the ear), variable output, variable tone, compression, directional microphone, and telephone coil.

This program allowed the user to store, edit, delete, and sort the aids as desired. The matching program asked the user for information concerning the client. The user can weight characteristics from mandatory (aid must have characteristics to be considered) through high, medium, and low need, to indifferent (characteristic not considered).

Hearing aids are ranked by order of match, with the company, model, and price included. While there are other characteristics by which hearing aids must be considered in the final analysis, Craig and Seigenthaler felt that the program provides preliminary information which can facilitate final hearing aid selection.

Donnelly

Donnelly (1982) also supported the use of the computer in the prescription process for hearing aid fitting. He suggested that the computer can select aids with the appropriate electroacoustic characteristics for individual clients. One of the problems he noted, which is well worth considering, is that using the computer to match hearing aids presupposes that the characteristics of all available aids are stored in the computer.

At present, hearing aid specifications are input by the user. The number of aids that could be potentially used in the selection process is sizable, and new models and model changes are ongoing. The amount of time that the user might spend just keeping track of the aids on the market could negate the efficiency of the match process. Donnelly suggested that a computer-based information network through which professionals who fit hearing aids could get on-line updates from the manufacturers would be the most advantageous. While some companies provide computer-based information on their own aids, there appears to be no move to provide a standard reporting format to which all companies would agree to input information.

Gans, VerHoef, and Berger

Another type of hearing aid selection by computer program was reported by Gans, VerHoef, and Berger (1983). Their program required the user to input air and bone conduction thresholds and uncomfortable loudnesses (UCLs). From this information, the computer made four calculations: predicted aided hearing levels, maximum gain requirements to achieve those levels, minimum desirable SSPL, and the maximum permissible SSPL. The eventual outcome of the program, including inserting values of commercial aids in a data bank for purposes of matching, was discussed previously. Gans et al. suggested that future efforts in computerizing the selection of hearing aids would include calculations of signal modification based on tubing length and diameters, venting of molds, effects of horns and filters, etc. They also suggested that the data from hearing aid fittings could be stored and later charateristics of successful versus unsuccessful fittings could be analyzed statistically. This, they felt, would lead to more predictable and precise hearing aid selection.

Preves

The potential of computer applications in the area of hearing aids may come through improving hearing aid design by incorporating a microprocessor in the aid itself. Preves (1982) stated that two of the most common problems in hearing aid fitting are "the detrimental effects of environmental noise on discrimination and the occurrence of acoustical feedback oscillation . . . in both high gain fittings as well as fittings utilizing large vents" (p. 15). He suggested that both problems might be alleviated by digital manipulation of the amplified signal. Digital filters have the capability of reducing the noise component of the signal while maintaining the integrity of the speech signal. In addition, through digital signal phase shift and other methods, acoustic feedback could be reduced, thereby permitting higher gain settings.

Preves pointed out that at the present time the equipment to accomplish such signal modification is too large to incorporate into existing hearing aid cases and requires more power than is currently available in hearing aid batteries. However, the minaturization of electronics contines to make strides in design efficiency. It is reasonable to look forward to a day in which digital manipulation of the signal will not only allow the above signal modification, but make dramatic improvements in frequency-gain characteristics, selective gain control, and control of temporal aspects of speech, i.e., sound compression and expansion.

Fitch

While the potential for electroacoustical matching and modification is impressive, there is a great deal more to fitting a hearing aid than the amplified signal itself. The behavioral considerations (how the individual responds to the hearing aid) is equally important to the quality of amplification. The author developed a program for evaluating appropriateness for hearing aid fitting (Fitch, 1983) by analyzing behavioral/environmental variables. Information was input to the computer regarding such things as the ability of the client to manipulate batteries, gain control, and switches, whether the client had worn a hearing aid before (and if so, the success of that fitting), the support that could be expected from the family, how realistic the client's expectations for the hearing aid were, and the client's motivation for improved understanding of conversation around him. These factors were weighted according to clinical observations of the user, and the computer calculated the perceived probability of success for fitting, i.e., excellent candidate for hearing aid fitting, good candidate, fair candidate, poor candidate, and client should not consider hearing aid fitting.

The computer did not compare electroacoustic characteristics in this program. The audiologist analyzed hearing loss contours and selected hearing aid models from which the client could choose. Most audiologists regularly use only a relatively few hearing aid choices and those choices are based on a combination of quality of craftsmanship, dependability, battery life, company return and repair policy, and price, in addition to electroacoustic characteristics. Most have variable tone and gain controls which allow for maximum signal shaping, so that amplification characteristics can be individualized for each client.

However, the final selection is not based on electroacoustic matching, it is based on client reaction to the aid. Amplification preference is very much a subjective evaluation and most professionals who fit hearing aids regularly will know the response characteristics of the aids well enough to choose ones that are "in the ball park." After that, it becomes a process of signal adjustment, venting, and selection of ear mold characteristics that will decide whether or not the fitting will be a successful one.

Other Programs

There are other programs available, and many more will emerge. Two very good resources for reviewing existing programs can be found in Sheeley (1984) and Jackson (1985). Some of these come as integrated programs which provide capability for inventory control as well as hearing aid selection (Glascoe, 1984b, c).

Summary—Hearing Aid Selection

In summarizing the utilization of the computer in hearing aid selection, it can be said that the computer is useful in making routine calculations and in matching characteristics of an individual hearing loss to the features of a set of hearing aids. However, the amount of time and effort required to input hearing aid specifications and keep that information updated limits a real gain in efficiency. Also, hearing aid fitting involves many factors that are not well adapted to quantification. Cosmetic considerations, personality characteristics, financial resources, and a host of other variables can play a critical role in hearing aid selection and must be accounted for in any practical hearing aid selection protocol.

In addition to the above, it must be recognized that there is no one clinical procedure now being used in hearing aid fitting that could be described as an industry standard. Until the process of hearing aid selection itself becomes a standardized, systematic, definable algorithm, there can be no meaningful computer-managed selection process. It has been stated before in this book that one of the most important benefits of the computer is that it forces the user to specify tasks in discrete, quantifiable steps. Perhaps this is the most advantageous aspect of the continuing efforts to develop computerized hearing aid selection procedures.

HEARING CONSERVATION PROGRAMS

There is no subfield in audiology that is as amenable to computer application as hearing conservation. Almost every phase of the hearing conservation program can utilize the computer to some degree.

Potential of the Computer

One of the primary needs in a hearing conservation program is a cost-effective means of testing large numbers of individuals. Several studies cited previously (Sparks, 1972; Wood, Wittich, & Mahaffey, 1973; Campbell, 1974; and others) have demonstrated the feasibility of computerized pure tone testing. Wood, Mahaffey, and Peters (1973) described a computerized testing procedure by which six men could be tested for pure tone determination concurrently using one computer.

The limitation of pure tone testing that has been noted in all studies is the hard-to-test client. In hearing conservation programs, however, most of the persons being tested have normal hearing and can respond appropriately in a structured testing paradigm. There are few hard-to-test clients so the computer can be heavily utilized for routine testing. In addition, computers can be programmed to recognize atypical response patterns. This means that the computerized test not only can screen for individuals who do not respond at expected hearing levels, but can also screen for individuals who demonstrate atypical response patterns. The ones who are identified as having atypical response patterns can then be tested face-to-face by an audiologist.

Analysis of hearing tests is a critical task in hearing conservation programs. The analysis is prescribed by federal regulations and requires that several calculations be performed on the data. First, the current guidelines from the *Federal Register* (U.S. Department of Labor, 1983) require that three frequencies (2K, 3K, and 4K) be averaged for each ear. The average of the most current test is compared to a baseline audiogram (audiogram obtained when the person began working for the industry or when the industry first initiated a hearing conservation program) to determine if a significant (standard) threshold shift has occurred. Before making this calculation, however, the guidelines require the audiologist to adjust the hearing level at each frequency for age. Tables are provided by the guidelines with different figures for males and females.

If the difference between the average of the adjusted critical frequencies for the current audiogram and the average of the adjusted critical frequencies for the baseline audiogram is greater than 10 dB, then the threshold shift is considered significant. When this occurs, the employee is retested to confirm the findings of the current audiogram. If the results are confirmed, then the employee and industry are informed that a significant threshold shift has occurred. At this point the audiologist administering the hearing conservation program may meet with the company and employee and take action to reduce the employee's exposure to noise.

While all of the calculations are reasonable and logical processes, the manual computation of them on large numbers of audiograms requires extraordinary amounts of time and invites errors. The computer can be programmed to perform the calculations with a significant savings in time and increased accuracy.

Existing Programs

One such computer management system (Smith & Borden, 1980) has been used to analyze over 100,000 audiograms. Using this system, hearing threshold test data was obtained by conventional testing methods and entered into the computer for analysis. One of the most common errors found by the authors of that program was the illegibility of manually recorded thresholds. To correct this problem, they devised optical scan cards, such as the kind often used in administering standardized examinations. The authors reported that other than an occasional smudge which the computer rejected, accuracy of data entry was greatly enhanced.

Smith and Borden (1980) also reported using the computer to generate various reports. Individual reports on each person tested were provided, with the results of both the baseline and the current audiogram included. A separate report identifying all of the persons tested who experienced significant threshold shifts was also generated. In addition, they provided a report of employees with hearing levels by type. The types A, B, C, D, and E related to sensitivity levels. Types A and B were normal hearing, and types C, D, and E indicated progressively more severe losses. Smith and Borden also calculated percentage hearing loss for individuals.

The author developed a computer-managed hearing conservation program that did essentially the same things as reported above (Fitch, 1984). Manually administered tests were entered into the computer for analysis. The computer generated an individual report, including the baseline audiogram, current audiogram, whether a significant threshold shift had occurred, hearing type, and identification of examiner, examinee, testing instrument, and testing instrument calibration date (see Fig. 23). A separate list of individuals with signficant threshold shifts was generated by the computer.

A list of all individuals in the hearing conservation program and lists of examinees by hearing type (as indicated in Smith & Borden's 1980 report) were provided to the industry. The author reported that the advantages of the computer-managed hearing conservation program are increased cost/time efficiency, improved accuracy of results, and attractive, standardized reporting formats (Fitch & Wold, 1984a, b). All of the above contribute to the satisfaction of the industry officials and make the administration of a hearing conservation program attractive to the practicing audiologist.

Summary—Hearing Conservation

Other commercially available programs exist (*Comsys*, 1983; *HEAR-CON*, 1984) and there are indications that many more will emerge. Large industries and institutions may develop their own, based on particular reporting requirements (Shipley, 1984). Because of the efficiency with which the computer can accomplish the calculations required and provide comprehensive reports, computer-managed hearing conservation programs will become a professional standard.

REHABILITATION

As indicated in the previous chapter, little has been done in the use of computers in rehabilitation audiology. The work that has been done is in the area of education of the deaf (see Suggested Readings, Chapter 10). There are other areas, however, which could utilize the computer.

One area would be hearing aid orientation. Much of the explanation on the care and treatment of a hearing aid could be accomplished through an interactive tutorial computer program. Progress through the orientation could be controlled by clients' responses, which indicate whether they

INDIVIDUAL HEARING RECORD

NAME: LONG, LOUIS L.   SEX: M DOB: 6/6/46
EMPLOYER: ACME TIN SMITHS   SSN: 666-66-6666
LOCATION: SHOP   SHIFT: 3RD

* *

DATE: 5/3/86   CURRENT TEST

                 500   1000   2000   3000   4000   6000   8000

RIGHT EAR   5   15   20   20   10   5   5
LEFT EAR   10   20   20   25   30   20   20

COMMENTS: NO PROBLEMS INDICATED.

* *

DATE: 3/1/85   BASELINE TEST

                 500   1000   2000   3000   4000   6000   8000

RIGHT EAR   5   10   15   20   5   5   5
LEFT EAR   10   20   15   25   25   15   15

COMMENTS: NO PROBLEMS INDICATED.

* *

AUDIOMETER (MAKE/MODEL)   CALIBRATION DATE
   BASELINE: TRACOR RA16   2/2/85
   CURRENT: TRACOR RA16   4/29/86

EXAMINER
   BASELINE: JLF/000-00-0000
   CURRENT: JLF/000-00-0000

HEARING STATUS

   NO SIGNIFICANT THRESHOLD SHIFT

   TYPE B AUDIOGRAM. HEARING WITH NORMAL LIMITS IN SPEECH FREQUENCIES
   IN BETTER EAR, BUT SOME TEST FREQUENCIES EXCEED 25 DB.
   THIS TYPE OF HEARING IS CONSIDERED WITHIN NORMAL LIMITS
   AND THE INDIVIDUAL SHOULD EXPERIENCE NO PROBLEMS
   IN COMMUNICATION.

Figure 23. Computer-managed hearing conservation individual report.

are understanding the material. Over time, this could save an office substantial time outlay.

Auditory training and Speech reading are also areas which could utilize computer management, especially if developed in conjunction with video disc capabilities. The computer could be programmed to present stimuli under a variety of conditions, ranging from the most ideal to the most difficult. A speech reading task could be presented with a speaker close up, and then at various distances depending on the proficiency of the client. Angle and lighting conditions could also be programmed to be under computer control.

Auditory training could be programmed using the same basic design. Speech could be presented under the best of conditions initially. Then, when the client demonstrates consistent comprehension, the conditions can be controlled for parameters such as intensity, distortion, and competing stimuli. The record-keeping procedures would assure good accountability for such a program.

As audiologists become more involved in the rehabilitation process, more programs for rehabilitation will emerge. Perhaps the process of computerizing procedures will encourage more systematic and accountability-conscious models.

OTHER ACTIVITIES IN AUDIOLOGY

The potential of computer-assisted instruction for the professional-in-training or the professional who desires continuing education has been recognized. Computer software which simulates the testing situation has been developed (Hood & Zimmerman, 1981; Glascoe, 1984a). These programs permit the user to practice administering audiometric tests that simulate the responses of individuals with different types of disorders. They allow the user to gain a great deal of experience and familiarity with the testing situation before actually testing clients.

A variety of other learning experiences can be programmed for students by integrating existing software with programs especially developed to meet particular needs (Lotterman, 1985). It is expected that as instructors become more familiar with computers, they will find audiology a field for which extensive computer-based learning opportunities can be developed.

CONCLUSION

The field of audiology was founded on a technological achievement, the electronic audiometer. The primary care provided by the field for rehabilition is amplification, founded on the technological capability which permits the use of minature circuitry in hearing aids. Given the technological orientation of the field, it is inevitable that the computer will become the basis for the hearing test of the future.

The computer will be used in all areas of audiological management. The most obvious uses have already become established, e.g., the development of database-managed hearing conservation programs and signal averaging for evoked auditory potentials. However, the potential of the computer to generate and control the acoustic signal through digital-to-analog conversion will lead to the use of stimuli that are much more complex. This will result in evaluation procedures that can test more parameters of hearing. Also, algorithms for many tests are amenable to artificial intelligence programming, so it is expected that more tests will be computer administered. This will result in more standardized and systematic testing procedures.

The final result will be audiologists who are capable of testing more people and testing them more quickly, thoroughly, and accurately. The computer will free audiologists to concentrate more on the client. They will have more data on which to base decisions and more time to devote to counseling and rehabilitation. Most audiologists would agree that that is the way it should be.

References

Campbell, R. (1974). Computer audiometry. *Journal of Speech and Hearing Research*, **17**, 134–140.

Comsys. (1983). Colorado Springs, CO: Comsys Corporation.

Craig, C., & Siegenthaler, B. (1981). Preliminary hearing aid selection by computer. *Hearing Aid Journal*, **34**, 8–9, 20.

Donnelly, K. (1982). Computer assisted hearing aid fitting. *Hearing Instruments*, **33**, 18–19.

Fitch, J. (1983). *Computerized hearing aid selection.* Gulfport, MS: Communicology Associates.

Fitch, J. (1984). *Computer managed hearing conservation.* Gulfport, MS: Communicology Associates.

Fitch, J., & Wold, J. (1984a). Computer managed hearing conservation. *National Hearing Conservation Association Newsletter*, August, 6–8.

Fitch, J., & Wold, J. (1984b). Hearing conservation programs for microcomputers. *Sound and Vibration*, **18**, 26–29.

Fritze, W. (1978). A computer-controlled binaural balance test. *Acta Otolaryngologica*, **86**, 89–92.

Gans, D., VerHoef, N., & Berger, K. (1983). Hearing aid selection by computer. *Hearing Instruments*, **34**, 17, 97.

Glascoe, G. (1984a). *Audiometer simulator.* State College, PA: Parrot Software.

Glascoe, G. (1984b). *Hearing aid manager.* State College, PA: Parrot Software.

Glascoe, G. (1984c). *Select a hearing aid.* State College, PA: Parrot Software.

Harris, J. (1980). A comparison of computerized audiometry by ANSI, Bekesy fixed-frequency, and modified ISO procedures in an industrial hearing conservation program. *Journal of Auditory Research*, **20**, 143–167.

HEARCON (1984). Austin, TX: Tracoustics.

Hertzano, T., Levitt, H., & Slosberg, R. (1979). Computer assisted hearing-aid selection. In Wolf, J., & Klatt, D. (Eds.), *Speech Communication Papers*, 97th Meeting of the Acoustical Society of America, New York, pp. 627–629.

Hood, R., & Zimmerman, H. (1981). Computerized audiometric programmable simulator. *Hearing Aid Journal*, **34**, 6, 20.

Jackson, C. (1985). *Computer applications in the hearing aid selection process*. Paper presented to the 15th Annual International Hearing Aid Seminar, San Diego.

Jerger, J., & Hayes, D. (1983). Latency of the acoustic reflex. *Archives of Otolaryngology*, **189**, 1–5.

Lotterman, S. (1985). *Development of computer assisted instruction in communication disorders*. Paper presented to the American Speech–Language–Hearing Foundation's Conference on Computers, January 1985, New Orleans.

MAB-100. (1984). Golden, CO: AND/OR Corporation.

Preves, D. (1982). The potential of computers and signal processing for hearing aids. *Hearing Instruments*, **33**, 15–16.

Ross, M. (1978). Hearing aid evaluation. In J. Katz (Ed.), *Handbook of clinical audiology* (pp. 524–542). Baltimore: Williams & Wilkins

Sakabe, N., Hirai, Y., & Itami, E. (1978). Modification and application of the computerized automatic audiometer. *Scandinavian Audiologica*, **7**, 105–109.

Sheeley, E. (1984). Microcomputers: Software directory and selected bibliography. *Ear and Hearing*, **5**, 371–374.

Shipley, T. (1984). Engineering software—develop in-house or purchase. *Sound and Vibration*, **18**, 22–24.

Skinner, P. (1978). Electroencephalic response audiometry. In J. Katz (Ed.), *Handbook of clinical audiology* (pp. 311–327). Baltomore: Williams & Wilkins.

Smith, C., & Borden, T. (1980). A new approach to industrial audiogram analysis. *Hearing Aid Journal*, **33**, 4, 47–49.

Sparks, D. (1972). The feasibility of computerized audiometry. *Journal of Auditory Research*, **12**, 62–66.

Stach, B., & Jerger, J. (1984). Acoustic reflex averaging. *Ear and Hearing*, **5**, 289–296.

U.S. Department of Labor, Occupational Safety and Health Administration. (1983). Occupational Noise Exposure, Hearing Conservation Amendment. *Federal Register*, **48**, 9738–9785.

Wittich, W., Wood, T., & Mahaffey, R. (1971). Computerized speech audiometric procedures. *Journal of Auditory Research*, **11**, 335–344.

Wood, T., Mahaffey, R., & Peters, R. (1973). A six-man computerized audiometer. *Journal of the Acoustical Society of America*, **54**, 338.

Wood, T., Wittich, W., & Mahaffey, R. (1973). Computerized pure-tone audiometric procedures. *Journal of Speech and Hearing Disorders*, **16**, 676–684.

12

Developing Software

GETTING INTO POSITION

The development of software that is clinically significant is not so much the emergence of a product as it is a process. Good software development comes through individuals working themselves into positions in which they can produce the software. Software reflects the personality and intelligence of the developer.

The computer is a medium through which clinicians can practice their profession more efficiently. It is also a means by which clinicians can provide others with a model program that can be replicated in any setting with a computer. Software developers in communication disorders did not evolve according to a master plan conceived in advance. Developers were first clinicians who began using the computer with their own case loads to achieve results better, faster, and/or more efficiently. The first persons to develop software did not do so with the thought of developing software which others in the field would use. They developed it for their own use, incorporating their own biases and individualizing it for specific settings.

As the price of hardware plummeted, more clinical institutions purchased computers. Clinicians began looking for software that would be of use in the clinical setting. They looked to the persons who had developed software for their own purposes to make that software available to the field. The need for clinically oriented software forced the early developers into choosing between providing the software through public domain or marketing it through normal communication disorders materials channels.

The demand was too great for developers to put material in the public domain (public domain software is software that has no copyright protection and for which there is no charge or minimal charge) and try to furnish copies to all who wanted them. The amount of time that it takes to create and test a program and the amount of support required when the software is distributed to the field are too demanding to continue for any length of time without financial resources. In addition, the cost of buying the computer hardware and software required to create programs is prohibitive, unless there is income to offset the expense.

The first successful developers were ones who persevered until their products reached the marketplace. They invested substantial amounts of time, energy, and money in their software. They were individuals with a healthy mixture of clinical proficiency, computer skill, and entrepreneurial spirit. It appears that this mixture can be achieved only by the person willing to "pay his dues" in learning the trade.

CLINICAL SKILLS

Without a doubt, the most important skill in developing clinically useful software is clinical proficiency. Developers must be intimately familiar with the clinical process that they are trying to program, and must be particularly understanding of the population for which they develop software. For example, clinicians working primarily with aphasics should develop software for that case load. In addition, clinicians must have something better to offer in the way of clinical processes if the software that they develop is to be significant.

Clinicians developing software must also have other skills. They must have the ability to stand back from the clinical process, analyse it, and understand how it operates. They must be able to formulate algorithms that solve clinical problems. In this regard, they must be able to translate clinical "insight" into a definable process which can be broken down into steps.

An example of insight in the clinical setting which can be translated into an algorithm is the ability that some clinicians possess when it comes to keeping young children on tasks. Clinicians who have insight into the behavior of young children cue on specific observable events, even though they themselves sometimes cannot verbalize what it is that they cue on. An example is response time. Clinicians who are good at keeping young children on task learn to anticipate when the children are starting to "fade" from the task. When this occurs, they change tasks or feedback strategies to get the child's attention back on task. Some of the definable cues that suggest that a child is "fading" are slower response rates, attempting to change topic/task, or poor eye contact.

As stated before, the clinician who is going to program a computer to duplicate what a clinician does must first be aware of all that a clinician does in the performance of duties. He must be able to break the clinical process into discrete units, or modules, which can be defined in terms of observable events. Before clinicians can develop computer software that will emulate clinical processes, they must be completely familiar with the clinical processes that are being emulated. There is no substitute for experience.

PROGRAMMING SKILLS

There are two primary approaches to developing clinical software. One approach is to hire a programmer, tell him what to program, and let him write the software; the second is to do it oneself. Either way, clinicians who want to develop software will find that they must know something about programming. Understanding programming, which is understanding a computer language, results in understanding how the computer does what it does. Therefore, it is critical for software developers to have considerable skill and knowledge regarding computer language, even though they may not do the actual programming themselves.

While there are several languages which can be used, the most common language used with communication disorders software is BASIC. This, plus the fact that BASIC is easy to learn, would make it the language of choice in most circumstances. However, if the person who wants to develop software is going to hire a programmer who will be using a different language, the clinician needs to be familiar with that language.

The author has only modest programming skills. However, he has found it more efficient, and less frustrating, to program himself rather than use a programmer. He found that programmers tend to approach tasks from the point of view of what is most efficient and logical for the machine. Clinical software, however, must be constructed from the point of view of what is most efficient and logical for the clinician and the client—and what is more efficient and logical for the machine is not always more efficient and logical for people.

It does not take a great deal of time to learn BASIC. In 2½ hours of training, most of the commands of the language can be learned. To be proficient in programming, however, requires a substantial investment in time and effort. Like writing stories, designing houses, or painting pictures, programming skills continue to grow and expand with experience.

The initial introduction to programming can be learned from a book, from a class at a college (or junior college or high school night class), or from a friend. Perhaps the most important of the above is the book. Many good reference books adorn the shelves of bookstores (and libraries) and through them almost any programming problem can be solved. Many have exemplary programs that you can enter into the computer from the keyboard. From studying how those programs work, beginners can develop ideas of how to adapt existing software to meet their own needs.

Learning to program comes primarily from learning the basic functions of the computer and then designing and building programs within those constraints. Access to a computer on a regular basis is probably the best asset that the beginner can have.

Another important source of help is resource persons. Almost every community today has many people who work with computer programming on some level. Cultivating acquaintances with these people and using them as resources can save significant time and frustration for the beginner. Be particularly alert to younger people who have good computer skills. They often take pride in being able to show older persons how to do things and may be the most patient of teachers. The author learned many of his programming strategies from individuals under 21 years of age.

User groups are popular, and through them the beginner can become acquainted with people who can help in many different areas. Computer user meetings often include presentations on topics of interest to the programmer: graphics, speech synthesis, computer file management, etc. Computer user groups often have a library of material which can be borrowed and some of which can be copied (public domain).

The last requirement for the beginner (and the advanced programmer) is magazines. There are excellent monthly journals that deal with specific computers and specific user needs. A selected list of these is found in Appendix D. The programmer should spend a good deal of time perusing the periodicals to keep abreast of new hardware and software, and for tips on innovative uses of the computer. Moreover, these magazines often have public domain software that can be keyed into the computer which can help the programmer to learn new concepts.

The author suggests that beginners learn programming by beginning to write clinically useful software while they are learning the language. Beginners should look for ways of incorporating new commands they have learned into programs that can be used clinically. Figure 24 is an example of a program that contains only a few commands, but could have some clinical usefulness as a counter.

```
50    HOME:VTAB10
60    PRINT "THIS IS A PROGRAM THAT KEEPS AN ONGOING"
70    PRINT:PRINT "RECORD OF PER CENT OF CORRECT"
80    PRINT:PRINT "RESPONSES."
90    PRINT:PRINT:PRINT:PRINT:INPUT "      (PRESS 'RETURN'
      TO CONTINUE)    ";X$
100   HOME:GOTO 190
110   VTAB 8:  PRINT "C, I, OR X?  ";:GET X$:PRINT X$
112   PRINT
120   IF X$="C" THEN C=C+1: GOTO 150
130   IF X$="X" THEN VTAB 8:PRINT "THAT'S
      IT!   ":END
140   IF X$<>"I" THEN 190
150   T=T+1
160   VTAB 15:PRINT "TOTAL ATTEMPTS:   ";T
170   PRINT:PRINT "TOTAL CORRECT:   ";C
180   P=C/T*100
190   IF P-INT(P)>.49999 THEN P=P+1
200   K=INT(P)
210   PRINT:PRINT "PERCENTAGE CORRECT:   ";K;" "
220   VTAB 22:PRINT "(C=CORRECT, I=INCORRECT, X=STOP)":
      VTAB 8:PRINT:GOTO 110
```

Figure 24.   Program for counting and reporting responses.

The beginner should start with small projects. The basic strategy should be to program small parts of the clincial process. As this is done, the programmer is building a set of modules, many of which can be applied to a wide variety of programs. The idea should be to first program the computer to do a small part of the clinical session, then a larger part, and thus continue expanding the role that the computer plays as far as possible.

Keep in mind that the computer does not replace the clinician. Once the computer has been programmed to do a task, that task is no longer a human task; it is a computer one. Humans should move on to things that only humans can do and leave the work that machines can do to machines.

PROGRAMMING MODULES

There are certain aspects of the clinical treatment process that are common to all clinical treatments and there are certain aspects of diagnostic protocols that are common to all diagnostic efforts. Treatment, for example, includes the following elements:

Stimulus Presentation. Responses may be elicited by pictures, written words, words generated from a speech synthesizer, and other means. Once the programmer has written a module for one program, that same module may be incorporated into a variety of software.

Response Mode. Keyboards, joysticks, touch screens, special switches, etc., all have special programming paradigms which must be learned when they are being used as input for software.

Judgment of Response. The input from the client must somehow be evaluated. Input from the keyboard, a joystick, voice analyzer, etc. must be compared against a model to determine appropriateness.

Reinforcement/Feedback. Most treatment programs include reinforcement and/or feedback. Feedback can be in the form of words on the screen, graphics, or words spoken through synthesizers and other external devices controlled by the computer. Once subroutines have been written, for one behavior, they can easily be inserted into other treatment programs.

Program Criteria. Decisions for presenting more difficult material, less difficult material, and branching to different material are a part of any treatment plan. These can be programmed into the computer in the form of counters which can keep track of total responses, correct responses, response latency, etc. Computations of percentage correct, consecutive correct responses, etc. can be made from this data and can be used in making decisions concerning clinical management.

Maintaining Records. Keeping results of treatment on diskettes requires understanding how computer file management functions. Computer file management systems can easily be adapted from one program to another.

Reporting Results. Formatting reports that are attractive and contain all the information desired in the form desired is critical to software with accountability features. Once report formats are established, they can be modified with relative ease to meet different clinical needs.

By computerizing the clinical process part by part, the beginning programmer can limit efforts to "do-able" projects on which future work can be built. The beginner who tries to program everything into early software development efforts is likely to meet with frustration that can be overwhelming. It is appropriate at this time to recall a recommendation made earlier in this book: the user should keep control of the computer rather than allow the computer to control the user.

PACKAGING THE PROGRAM

Most clinical software programs contain several components. As components are constructed they can be incorporated into one large program, or they can be stored as separate programs which can be called from the disk via a master program. Some software may be divided into programs on several different disks. The choice should be based on what is most efficient for the user.

Another part of the packaging process is deciding how to teach the user how to interact with the program. An accompanying set of written instructions is probably the most common procedure. However, the most palatable method, and one that seems to be gaining widespread favor, is to include a tutorial program with the program disk itself. In this manner, the user is led through the program step by step by the computer. Tutorial programs can simply be instructions printed on the screen, or they can be interactive.

FIELD TESTING

One of the most critical parts of the development process is the field test of the material by the developer. Developers should take each module as it is developed and work with it in clinical settings themselves. Ideas that seem great initially are sometimes quickly found to be critically flawed. Obvious types of programming errors should not get in the field test beyond the field test by developers themselves.

Developers should carry out a field test on their own material by subjecting it to all of the errors they can conceive that could be made by a person in the field. In other words, they should see if they can make the program "crash." Building in error-trapping routines that recognize, and instruct the user how to correct, various errors is called affectionately "idiot proofing" (for obvious reasons). Programs less susceptible to crashing because of an input error by the user will find more widespread acceptance.

Software developers cannot always find the weak parts of their own programs. This is because they are so familiar with the program that they may compensate for the limitations without realizing it. Considering this, software needs as much outside review as possible. The first level of the outside review should be a trusted colleague, one who will give the software a completely honest review and look for ways to improve it. This reviewer should diligently try to find all of the things that can cause the program not to work the way it should. Since this requires a good deal of time and effort, the reviewer must be someone who is well disposed toward the developer. The results of the initial field test by an educated user is invaluable in revising the program.

The last phase of field testing is to give the program to users who are unsophisticated in software usage. Experienced computer users sometimes miss major flaws simply because they know computers and will not make the "dumb" or obvious errors. Well-written software should protect against even obvious errors if it is to be useful to people who have limited computer backgrounds.

Throughout the field test, the theme is "continually debug, debug, debug, and then debug some more." Debugging is a matter of not only correcting errors in the program, but also making changes that make the program work faster, more efficiently, or easier for the user. Clinical programs should be tested hundreds of times in the field test before they are considered candidates for distribution. One program that the author developed was administered in over 1800 treatment sessions before one small, minor error (that happened to cause the program to crash and data to be lost) was found. The odds of a user making that particular error were 2000 to 1. However, even that is not acceptable if it can be prevented.

Field tests should be documented as much as possible. Supporting material containing test results that have been generated, analyzed, organized and written into understandable form will give the software more credibility to the clinician in the field.

SELF-PUBLISHING VERSUS COMMERCIAL PUBLISHING

Once software has been developed, field tested, and found to be clinically useful, the developer must select a strategy for making it available to the field. Basically that can be reduced to two choices. The developer can agree to distribution by a commercial publisher, or the developer can become a publisher.

There are two major advantages to self-publishing. First, self-publishing gives developers more control over how the final product will look and to whom it will be marketed. Second, developers publishing their own material receive the total profit from a sale rather than a percentage.

However, the developer who decides to self-publish must be prepared to learn business skills. There are general business procedures such as accounts receivable and payable, general ledger, mailing lists, invoices, return policies, advertising, design, and packaging and other management skills that need to be learned for a software package to be successfully marketed. Making arrangements for copy protection, printing documentation, and package design require, at least the first time around, a great deal of time and effort.

Before making the decision to become one's own publisher, developers should determine if they have the time, motivation, and desire to learn, and engage in, the business world. Equally important, since publishing material requires that money be spent before the product is sold, a substantial amount of capital may be needed. The success of a software marketing venture is only partially dependent on the quality of the product. The rest depends on how well it is produced and marketed.

Having a publisher develop and market a software product has the advantage of taking less of the developers' time, requiring less capital outlay, and removing the necessity of learning the publishing business. Because many developers are employed, and prefer to write programs rather than become business people, this may be the most expedient avenue for the majority.

However, having a publisher produce and market the software does not solve all of the developer's problems. Developers should realize that there are considerations that must be addressed in working with publishers. The contract between a publisher and a developer should be carefully read, and understood, by the developer. Developers should be aware of what is required of them during the publishing process. Contracts may require that the developer make program modifications as dictated by the company. Contracts may require the developer to present clinics or workshops on the material—sometimes with compensation, sometimes without compensation. The developer may also be asked to give first options on new material developed to the publisher. Finally, the developer must agree on the royalty rate. Royalty rates, that is, payment to the developer by the publisher, may range from 10 to 30% of the sale price, depending on how much product modification and development is required of the publisher. Obviously, it is important that developers choose publishers with established records of integrity and capability in materials distribution.

CONCLUSION

Developing a software product that is clinically useful is a formidable task. It requires individuals with clinical skills, an understanding of computers, and considerable patience and perseverance. For the product to be successful in the field, it must do something better, faster, or easier than it is done without a computer. These things occur only through the efforts of individuals who have spent a great deal of time learning their trade.

The rewards for those who do persevere can be outstanding. Successful programs bring recognition, financial compensation, and the satisfaction of seeing one's own work replicated in many settings. A good software package is not only good for the developer; it is of course good for the people in the field. By making life a little easier for those who use it, the developer may receive the greatest reward of all.

13

The Future

REASONS TO CONSIDER THE FUTURE

It is reasonable to ask the question "why look into the future?" Aside from being a fun kind of mental exercise, does thinking about the future have any real significance? The response to that is a resounding *yes*. Looking into the future is as important as any task faced in professional life. It meets several critical needs for growth of the professional, and of the profession. Predicting the general direction of the future of a discipline is not terribly difficult. The accuracy of predictions is approximately logarithmically related to the time span for which the prediction is made. The further into the future the prediction is made, the less likely it is to be accurate. However, even if the predictions are not particularly accurate, the exercise is a healthy one.

First, it is healthy because predicting the future is done by making logical inferences based on current practices. This requires that the individual making the predictions study current practices. The process of examining what exists, in view of identifying critical elements that are likely to endure and become enhanced, makes for a professional who is current in the field. Second, thinking of the future is usually done in scenarios that are not locked into one mode of thinking. It is a game of "if this happens, then what changes could it possibly bring about?" The number of different scenarios that can be envisioned by asking this question is limited only by the time that an individual wishes to spend on the exercise.

This type of mental exercise encourages flexibility and consideration of alternatives. This seems particularly important to professionals in communication disorders because training programs in the field have their roots in tightly structured academic programs which are designed to meet tightly structured credentialing requirements. That type of training tends to promote rigidity in thinking.

Future thinking is akin to putting a puzzle together. Individual pieces of the puzzle can be tested in different configurations to see their effect on the whole. However, since the future does not exist yet, there are always pieces missing from the "what if" picture. These pieces have to be created in the mind of the person participating in the exercise to make the picture complete. This promotes creativity, another healthy trait that does not always find encouragement in training programs.

Another reason to consider the future is to prepare professionals for the future before it arrives, to avoid future shock. Professionals can cope with the future better if they have some idea of what it holds. They will be better prepared if they have time to develop the skills which will be necessary in the future. Finally, and perhaps most importantly, professions as a whole need to consider the future from the point of view that much of what the future holds is determined by what the members of the profession want it to be. By looking at the alternatives and choosing to promote those which appear to have the most potential for enhancing the profession, members can to a great degree shape their own future. Participation in professional activites and active communication between fields, and between subdisciplines within the field, can influence the course of the profession.

CONSIDERING OTHER INFLUENCES

Looking into the future also forces the professional to consider what is happening in other disciplines. Two major forces which shape today's society and which will continue to be dominant influences in the future are the telephone and television. Telephones and television altered the primary means by which information was transmitted in society.

Before the telephone the primary means of conveying personal and business information was through the mail. Now a great percentage of the population prefers to call to visit with friends or conduct business rather than write letters. It permits immediate two-way dialogue which enhances the communication act immeasurably. In addition, postal rates and the cost of preparing a business letter have risen to the point that it is sometimes as cost efficient to call as it is to send a letter.

There will undoubtedly be more innovations which will promote the use of the telephone. One, of course, is the computer itself. The interface of the computer and the telephone permits the exchange of information with a high rate of efficiency. The greater the amount of information that is sent, the more cost efficient it will be to send it from computer to computer over the telephone lines.

Television has displaced magazines and newspapers as the major dispenser of public information. More people watch television than read books or magazines for news, information, and entertainment. The interface of the computer with television will enhance the popularity of television to an even greater degree than it already enjoys.

In the future, computers will give the user a means of interacting with television programming. The use of the computer–television interface for such mundane tasks as shopping is already being tested in the United States. Television companies are now considering shows that will permit the viewer to participate in the program, to the point of determining how a show will end.

Political scientists are considering the television–computer interface as a means of rediscovering democracy (Laver, 1980). After observing a debate on television, the viewers can vote, or give their legislators input on how to vote, on issues before Congress. The capability of the computer for processing large amounts of data in small periods of time could enable millions to vote on an issue in the time that it now takes the legislators to vote (Laver, 1980).

OTHER FORCES AT WORK

Aside from the technology, there are other developments which the author feels will increasingly shape the future of professionals in communication disorders. One is the orientation of the profession as a whole. The author feels that in the early history of communication disorders, the basic orientation of the clinician was to approach the profession as an "art." In the model of medicine, however, he feels that there is a growing tendency in communication disorders to approach the field as a "science."

Much of the reorientation is out of necessity. Just as patients who need medical treatment prefer hospitals with the latest technology, individuals with communication disorders will want the services of agencies which are more current in their approach to treatment, and the status of technology within the agency is (whether accurate or not) viewed by the outsider as a major indicator of how current the agency is in its overall approach to treatment.

Another factor to consider is the technology associated with the computer itself. The generic term *computer* will probably give way to a plethora of technology that will include the basic present-day electronic processing capability, but have other names and be designed for special purposes. Just as the first gas-powered vehicle, the automobile, gave rise to compacts, limousines, sedans, convertibles, sports cars, trucks (semi, pick-up, dump, refrigerated, tanker), vans, four-wheelers, station wagons, and so on, the generic computer will spawn generations of electronic instruments which will increasingly be designed to meet the needs of specific populations.

The author believes that understanding the future of a profession is found in understanding the future of society as a whole. Developments in the profession will not follow paths completely unique to the rest of society. It is important that, as a profession, members continue to be aware of significant developments in other disciplines. In all likelihood, they will be the next significant developments in their own field.

A DAY AT THE CLINIC—YEAR 2010

Mail Call

The clinician of the future will begin the day in much the same way as today's clinician—by checking the mailbox. However, instead of actual boxes, the mailbox will be electronic. The electronic mailbox will contain the same type of information that is now deposited in mailboxes, but there will be differences. First, there will be letters and communications from all over the country (or world for that matter) in the mailbox when the day starts. This will be because phone rates are cheaper in the late evening hours. Mail will be compiled during the day and sent in batches at night. The computer will be programmed to send and receive mail according to instructions put into the computer by the user. All of the sorting and sending will be done in the evening with no human supervision needed. This will eliminate the lag time of agency mail rooms and the postal service. All of the things that are presently sent through the mail will come this way. Only three-dimensional material, or material that must be sent physically intact, will go through the mail system as it is now known.

As the individual reads the mail, answers can be composed on the word processor. A simple key stroke at the end will send the response back to the sender (through the return address already in the computer). Thus, the "float" time in responding to mail will be reduced dramatically. Of course, the receiver will have the option of saving the mail electronically, or even printing a hard copy on the printer. However, if the communication is not something that needs to be kept, it can be discarded electronically. "Junk mail" will no longer go in the wastebasket; it will simply be erased from memory.

Inter- and Intraoffice Communication

After viewing mail from outside the agency, the professional will look for electronic memorandums from within. Instead of having a copy sent to each individual in the agency, a memorandum will be put on the computer and directed to all of the mailboxes. A supervisor can put a memorandum in the box early in the morning (or before leaving the previous day) and be sure each member of the staff will get it at the beginning of the day. Again, these notices can be stored or hard copies made from them, but they can also be erased. File thirteen will be an electronic phantom and routing slips will become a topic of discussions that begin "I remember when. . . ."

Documents will be transmitted electronically between agencies as well. Mailing lists will be used for electronic mail just as they are now used for sending correspondence through the postal service. For example, a state education agency could leave an electronic memorandum for everyone on its mailing list. However, unlike the mailing list of today which requires some human processing for each piece, electronic mail can be sent to as many agencies as desired with no more effort than is now required to send one piece of mail. This will encourage greater dissemination of information, and also create large amounts of mail to process. Perhaps the computer will then be programmed to screen incoming mail for important versus "junk" mail.

During the day information will be transmitted in a similar manner within the agency. Documents for the secretary to process will be sent electronically. Editing can be done on the word processor by both the writer and the secretary before the final product is readied for mail.

One of the chief duties of the secretary will be to assemble the day's work for the evening transmission. The amount of document preparation by secretaries will be reduced substantially as individuals will do more of their own word processing, leaving the secretary the task of checking and formatting the final output of the document.

Diagnosis and Treatment

After reading and responding to the morning mail, the clinician may, for example, conduct treatment with an aphasia group. Six to eight clients come in for individual and group work. During the first half of the session the clinician works with one or two at a time while the rest work on individual lessons at computers. The second half of the session is devoted to counseling the group as a whole. After the session the clinician reviews the results of the individual treatments on the computer and enters information for the next day's lesson.

The clinician of the future may then prepare for a diagnostic case that is scheduled. This starts by a review of the records, which have been sent electronically. Perhaps this is a case that has a disorder with which the clinician is not familiar. Instead of going to the library to collect information, the clinician will call the library and conduct a search of information on the disorder through the computer–telephone interface. After finding several pertinent references, the references can be entered from the library computer to the clinician's computer and stored in memory or printed out on paper. Libraries from anywhere in the world can be searched and the needed information made available in minutes. Complete books can be sent, and printed in minutes on the agency's laser printer.

While the clinician is completing preparations for the diagnostic session, the client arrives and is interviewed by the computer. Standard case history information is entered, after which the computer asks the client questions. The interview is adaptive in nature; that is, the questions asked by the computer depend on the response of the client to previous questions. When the computer learns that the individual being seen was born with a cleft palate or hearing loss, it will ask questions to explore that phase of the client's history. This will save time from the normal intake interview process and yield more meaningful information.

During the diagnostic session most of the activities will incorporate the use of the computer. Articulation tests will consist of having the client say words, or sentences, into a microphone. The sample will be stored (in digital form) and the acoustic characteristics analyzed. A report will be generated with distinctive feature analysis, developmental analysis, analysis of error patterns with suggestions for possible etiology, and recommendations for treatment. Information on performance will be based on statistical analysis so that the term *within normal limits* will have a much more significant meaning than it has now.

Receptive language will be measured by the client taking a computer-based test, the construction of which will probably differ very little from what is available today in paper form. The testing will be adaptive, however, with the computer presenting more difficult or less difficult test items based on the responses of the client. When the test is completed, it will be instantaneously scored and analyzed for error patterns, and a report generated with percentiles, standard deviations, and other pertinent information. It will suggest other possible tests, indicate suspected etiologies, and recommend possible treatment protocols and prognosis.

Expressive language will be analyzed using tests very similar to those of today. However, the client will speak into a microphone and the computer will perform the analysis in a manner similar to that indicated with the articulation test. One such test might ask the client to look at pictures on the monitor and respond to the question "what is happening in the picture?" As the client speaks, the computer analyzes responses and presents more pictures based on the input already obtained.

At the same time that the linguistic analysis is being done, an analysis of voice—pitch, intensity, and quality—is also being performed by the computer using the same sample. Fluency patterns will also be quantified by analyzing the same sample for temporal characteristics of the signal.

At the end of the diagnostic session, the computer will generate a report on each of the areas tested and unify it into draft form for an overall report. The clinician will edit the report and discuss the findings with the client. The time saved during the diagnostic session by utilizing the computer can be spent with the client. A copy of the report can be given to the client at that time and sent electronically to any source that needs a copy of it. Again, the float time of information exchange will be significantly reduced.

After the diagnostic session, our future clinician may meet with a group for articulation treatment. However, instead of working as a group, each individual goes to a learning station and follows a computer-managed program. The client follows directions (on screen if he can read, voice commands from speech synthesis if not) and makes responses into a microphone. An acoustic analysis is performed and immediate feedback provided on the accuracy of response. If the individual is in the early stages of learning the sound, the computer will provide feedback for progressively more accurate productions. A variety of elicitation techniques will be used to obtain maximum generalization. The computer has records on each individual and can select treatment not only on what is happening at the present session, but in view of the total treatment plan.

Several individuals can be monitored by the clinician at one time. Programs may have built-in signals, such as beeps or flashing lights, to signal the clinician that an individual needs help. At the end of the session the computer will print a cumulative report which the client can keep for his own records.

Later in the day perhaps a hearing-impaired child is scheduled for aural rehabilitation. A video disc–computer interface presents speech reading and auditory discrimination exercises. Distance, lighting, and angle for speech reading are varied to simulate actual listening conditions. Speech is controlled for intensity and quality, and background noise is added to simulate actual listening conditions. The computer monitors the performance and changes stimulus parameters to meet the individual's performance needs. After getting the child started on the computer, the clinician can meet with the parent(s) and participate in a counseling program.

Professional Development

Maybe this is the day that our clinician of the future participates in professional development. To maintain certification status in the future, the author suggests that clinicians will be required to follow professional development plans filed with the credentialing agency. The professional development plan may work as follows. The clinician calls the agency computer and reviews the professional development plan. The computer then indicates areas of professional knowledge and skills that need to be updated. The clinician selects the area with which he wants to work this day and the computer calls up a computer-assisted instruction module that will present the information.

While the clinician participates in the learning experience, the computer scores the answers and at the end of the exercise provides a report on how the clinician has done in comparison to other clinicians with comparable training and experience. The information is logged back to the agency computer where his professional development file is updated.

Requisitions

Later in the day our clinician learns that there is some money in the budget for upgrading clinical equipment and supplies. The clinician calls a supplier to gain access to an electronic catalog, which lists all of the available materials, in the same manner that paper catalogs now do the job. He can call demonstration materials on the screen to see how things look and work.

When the clinician finds something he wants to purchase, he places the order through the computer–telephone interface. If the material is computer software or something that can be printed on paper, it will be entered into his computer at that moment so the clinician will have the material available immediately. After receipt of the material has been certified, the company computer will update the agency's account to reflect the purchase. The clinician will not have to deal with the delays of purchase orders, or the postal system, unless he is ordering materials that cannot be transmitted electronically.

Next our clinician may decide to update the clinic's library. Another electronic catalog with a listing of publishers will provide the vehicle for making this purchase. As above, he will be able to review the material electronically and when he is ready to purchase documents, it will be done on-line with the computer. The documents that he purchases can be received by his computer and printed using a laser printer in a matter of minutes. The material will also be stored electronically so that utility programs to search for specific information may be used. Since the material now belongs to the clinician, pages or even chapters can be rewritten by him to meet specific needs. The clinician may even want to take several chapters from different books to put them together to make one that has exactly the information that he wants and that is organized in just the fashion he desires.

Electronic catalogs/shopping will also be available for equipment, furniture, professional development materials, visuals aids, etc. As the clinician is ordering, the budget figure is being updated by the computer. Most likely, beeps will sound and messages flash to inform the clinician when he has spent the available funds.

High Touch

In the afternoon there will be a variety of activities which will be available to the clinician to provide opportunities for self-improvement. Some groups will emphasize physical well being with exercise programs. Others will function as present-day encounter groups to help individuals understand themselves and the people around them better. There will be activities on coping with stress, developing interpersonal communication skills, establishing efficient work habits, and others. As the profession moves to *high tech* applications, *high touch* (or humanistic) activities will emerge (Naisbitt, 1982). We cannot yet conceive the depth and breadth of opportunity for self-realization that will be available in the future.

The activities above will be an integral part of his the clinician's day because in the technological world of the future, a higher value will be placed on individuals as people. Management will recognize this and provide opportunities for individuals to develop themselves as people. This will not be done totally out of humanitarian concern, but because employers will find that the individual who is healthier, happier, and more confident is more efficient, performs his job better, and is less prone to absenteeism.

Day's End

In the same manner as the present-day clinician, the clinician of the future will check the mailbox before going home to see if there are any last-minute concerns. He will check the night transmissions he has prepared during the day and make last-minute changes. He will probably bring up the schedule for the next day on the monitor to see what challenges he will face. Then, recognizing quitting time through the internal clock, the computer will bid our clinician a pleasant good night and remind him where he is to meet a friend for dinner.

PREPARING FOR THE FUTURE

It is the author's impression that there need be little anxiety on the part of the clinician concerning the impact of the computer. The changes that will occur will be gradual. Each development will have to prove itself in many settings before it is accepted by professionals in the field. During the time it will take for this to occur, clinicians will have many opportunities available to learn about computers. If they avail themselves of those opportunities, and keep informed about how newly emerging software can be integrated in their own settings, the computer will become a part of their daily lives in a very natural way.

Another point is that computer software is becoming more and more user friendly. Tutorials that teach the clinician how to use the software will be included in the software package, so that training will be an integral part of any new software package. All in all, it should be a comfortable transition for the field.

Another very positive aspect of the future is that the inclusion of the computer into clinical processes will increase employment opportunities for professionals in communication disorders. There will be a need for professionals who can develop software packages and others who can design training packages. There will be a need for coordinators at local, state, and regional levels to review newly emerging software, disseminate information, and coordinate acquisitions. The author estimates that computer-related employment will increase the number of professional employment opportunities in communication disorders by 5–10%.

CONCLUDING STATEMENT

Preparation for the future will be an individual matter. Some clinicians will be affected more, some less. A few will focus their energies on the opportunities with computers and make it central to their careers. Most will incorporate it as just another tool which helps them become better professionals. The end result will be professionals who can more efficiently provide better services to more people. And for a professional, that is the bottom line.

References

Laver, M. (1980). *Computers and social change*. London and New York: Cambridge University Press.

Naisbitt, J. (1982). *Megatrends: Ten new directions transforming our lives*. New York: Warner Books.

Appendix A: Utility Programs for Communication Disorders

(The programs in Appendix A are written in Applesoft BASIC. They will work "as is" on Apple and Apple-compatible computers. Minor revisions will be needed for use with BASIC in other computers.)

```
100  REM   PROGRAM FOR COMPUTING CHRONOLOGICAL AGE
110  HOME : VTAB 10
120  PRINT "PROGRAM FOR COMPUTING CHRONOLOGICAL AGE"
130  VTAB 20: INPUT "(PRESS 'RETURN' TO CONTINUE)";X$
140  HOME : VTAB 6
150  PRINT "BIRTHDATE (USE NUMBERS ONLY):"
160  PRINT : HTAB 10: INPUT "MONTH:  ";MB
170  IF MB > 12 THEN 160
180  PRINT : HTAB 10: INPUT "DAY:    ";DB
190  IF DB > 31 THEN 180
200  PRINT : HTAB 10: INPUT "YEAR:   ";YB
210  IF YB > 82 THEN 200
220  HOME : VTAB 6
230  PRINT "TODAY'S DATE (USE NUMBERS ONLY):"
240  PRINT : HTAB 10: INPUT "MONTH:  ";TM
250  IF TM > 12 THEN 240
260  PRINT : HTAB 10: INPUT "DAY:    ";TD
270  IF TD > 31 THEN 260
280  PRINT : HTAB 10: INPUT "YEAR:   ";TY
290  IF TY < 83 THEN 280
300  IF TD > = DB GOTO 320
310  TM = TM - 1:TD = TD + 30
320  PD = TD - DB
330  IF TM > = MB GOTO 350
340  TY = TY - 1:TM = TM + 12
350  PM = TM - MB
360  PY = TY - YB
370  IF PD < 31 THEN 390
380  PM = PM + 1:PD = PD - 31
390  IF PM < 12 GOTO 410
400  PY = PY + 1:PM = PM - 12
410  HOME : VTAB 8
420  PRINT "THE PERSON'S AGE IS:"
430  PRINT : PRINT "      ";PY;" YEARS, ";PM;" MONTHS, ";PD;" DAYS"
440  VTAB 20: PRINT "PRESS 'Y' TO COMPUTE ANOTHER AGE."
450  PRINT : INPUT "PRESS ANY OTHER KEY TO END PROGRAM  ";X$
460  IF X$ = "Y" GOTO 140
470  END


90   REM    PROGRAM TO KEEP ONGOING DATA
100  HOME : VTAB 10
110  PRINT "THIS IS A PROGRAM THAT KEEPS AN ONGOING"
120  PRINT : PRINT "TABULATION OF PER CENT OF CORRECT"
130  PRINT : PRINT "RESPONSES."
140  PRINT : PRINT : PRINT : INPUT "     (PRESS 'RETURN' TO CONTI
     NUE)    ";X$
150  HOME : GOTO 280
160  VTAB 8: PRINT "C, I, OR X?  ";: GET X$: PRINT X$
170  PRINT
180  IF X$ = "C" THEN C = C + 1: GOTO 210
190  IF X$ = "X" THEN  VTAB 8: PRINT "THAT'S IT!  ": END
200  IF X$ < > "I" THEN 280
210  T = T + 1
220  VTAB 15: PRINT "TOTAL ATTEMPTS:  ";T
230  PRINT : PRINT "TOTAL CORRECT:  ";C
240  P = C / T * 100
250  IF P - INT (P) > .49999 THEN P = P + 1
260  K = INT (P)
270  PRINT : PRINT "PERCENTAGE CORRECT:  ";K;" "
280  VTAB 22: PRINT "(C=CORRECT, I=INCORRECT, X=STOP)"
290  VTAB 8: GOTO 160
```

```
90   REM      HEADS AND TAILS
100  HOME : VTAB 8
110  I = 4
120  V = 0:U = 0
130  PRINT "THIS IS A GAME OF HEADS AND TAILS."
140  PRINT : PRINT "MATCH WHAT I'M THINKING AND WIN."
150  PRINT : PRINT : PRINT "PICK A NUMBER BETWEEN 1-100 TO"
160  PRINT : INPUT "RANDOMIZE GAME:  ";I
170  PRINT : PRINT : PRINT "WHEN YOU ARE READY TYPE 'Y'  ";: GET X$
180  IF X$ = "Y" GOTO 200
190  GOTO 170
200  HOME
210  VTAB 6
220  PRINT "HEADS OR TAILS?  (H/T) ";
230  GET X$
240  PRINT
250  VTAB 12: PRINT "YOU    ME"
260  Z$ = "T"
270  IF  RND (I) > .50 THEN Z$ = "H"
280  PRINT : PRINT : PRINT X$;"      ";Z$
290  IF X$ = Z$ GOTO 330
300  U = U + 1
310  PRINT : PRINT "TOO BAD! YOU LOSE!"
320  GOTO 350
330  PRINT : PRINT "GREAT! YOU WIN!   "
340  V = V + 1
350  PRINT : PRINT : PRINT "YOU=";V;"     ME=";U
360  IF U = 10 GOTO 420
370  IF V = 10 GOTO 420
380  VTAB 8: PRINT "                          "
390  VTAB 10: PRINT "                         "
400  VTAB 6: HTAB 24: PRINT " "
410  GOTO 210
420  HOME : VTAB 10
430  PRINT "FINAL SCORE:"
440  PRINT : PRINT : PRINT "   YOU=";V
450  PRINT : PRINT "   ME=";U
460  PRINT : PRINT : PRINT "WANT TO PLAY AGAIN? (Y/N)  ";: GET X$
470  IF X$ = "Y" THEN 100
480  IF X$ < > "N" THEN 420
490  PRINT : PRINT : PRINT "END OF GAME.": END


90   REM     PROGRAM TO CALCULATE PERCENTAGE
100  HOME : VTAB 8: PRINT "THIS IS A SIMPLE PROGRAM THAT"
110  PRINT : PRINT "CALCULATES PERCENTAGE."
120  PRINT : PRINT : PRINT : PRINT : PRINT : INPUT "    (PRESS '
     RETURN' TO CONTINUE)   ";X$
130  HOME : VTAB 7
140  INPUT "TOTAL RESPONSES:  ";X
150  PRINT : PRINT : INPUT "TOTAL CORRECT:   ";Y
160  XY = Y / X
170  XY = 100 * XY
180  X1 = XY -  INT (XY)
190  IF X1 > .49999 THEN XY =  INT (XY) + 1
200  XY =  INT (XY)
210  VTAB 15: PRINT "PER CENT=";XY
220  VTAB 20: INPUT "WANT TO DO ANOTHER? (Y/N)  ";Z$
230  IF Z$ = "N" THEN  HOME : VTAB 10: PRINT "END OF PROGRAM   ": END
240  IF Z$ = "Y" THEN 130
250  GOTO 220
```

C1

```
100   REM "DAYS 'TIL CHRISTMAS!!!"
110   DIM DT(12)
120   HOME : VTAB 10
130   FOR I = 1 TO 12: READ DT(I): NEXT I
140   PRINT "PROGRAM FOR FINDING # OF DAYS"
150   PRINT : PRINT "UNTIL CHRISTMAS."
160   VTAB 22: INPUT "     (PRESS 'RETURN' TO CONTINUE)      ";X$
170   HOME : VTAB 10
180   INPUT "MONTH (1-12):  ";M
190   IF M > 12 THEN 180
200   PRINT : INPUT "DAY (1-31):     ";D
210   IF D > 31 THEN 200
220  D1 = 359 - D - DT(M)
230   IF M = 12 THEN  IF D > 25 THEN D1 = D1 + 365
240   PRINT : PRINT : PRINT : PRINT : PRINT "NUMBER OF DAYS 'TIL CHRISTMAS
      =";D1
250   VTAB 22: INPUT "WANT TO DO ANOTHER DATE? (Y/N)  ";X$
260   IF X$ = "Y" THEN 170
270   IF X$ < > "N" THEN 250
280   HOME : VTAB 22: PRINT "END OF PROGRAM": END
290   DATA  0,31,59,90,120,151,181,212,243,273,304,334
```

```
90   REM    GAME OF ROCK, PAPER, SCISSORS
100  HOME : VTAB 8: PRINT "THIS IS THE GAME ROCK, PAPER, SCISSORS"
105  PRINT : PRINT : INPUT "PICK A NUMBER BETWEEN 1 AND 100.  ";Z
135  HOME
140  VTAB 8: PRINT "ROCK, PAPER OR SCISSORS? (R,P,S)  ";
150  GET X$
152  IF X$ = "S" THEN 160
154  IF X$ = "R" THEN 160
156  IF X$ < > "P" THEN 135
160  Y =  RND (Z)
170  IF Y < .33 THEN W$ = "S"
180  IF Y > .33 THEN W$ = "R"
190  IF Y > .66 THEN W$ = "P"
192  IF X$ = "S" THEN U$ = "SCISSORS"
194  IF X$ = "R" THEN U$ = "ROCK    "
196  IF X$ = "P" THEN U$ = "PAPER   "
204  IF W$ = "S" THEN V$ = "SCISSORS"
206  IF W$ = "R" THEN V$ = "ROCK    "
207  IF W$ = "P" THEN V$ = "PAPER   "
208  PRINT : PRINT : PRINT "YOUR CHOICE:  ";U$
209  IF W$ = X$ THEN 230
210  U = U + 1
220  GOTO 240
230  V = V + 2
240  PRINT : PRINT "MY CHOICE:  ";V$
245  PRINT : PRINT "ME=";U;"     YOU=";V
246  IF U = 10 THEN 260
247  IF V = 10 THEN 260
250  GOTO 140
260  HOME : VTAB 10
270  PRINT "FINAL SCORE:"
280  PRINT : PRINT : PRINT "  YOU=";V
290  PRINT : PRINT "   ME=";U
300  VTAB 20: PRINT "    WANT TO PLAY AGAIN? (Y/N)   ";
310  GET X$
320  IF X$ < > "Y" THEN 330
325  U = 0:V = 0: GOTO 100
330  IF X$ < > "N" THEN 300
335  GOTO 300
340  PRINT : PRINT : PRINT "END OF GAME": END
```

Appendix B: List of Software Companies with Software for Professionals in Communication Disorders

SOFTWARE COMPANIES-COMMUNICATION DISORDERS

Laureate Learning Systems, Inc.
One Mill Street
Burlington, VT 05401

Communication Skill Builders
3130 N. Dodge Blvd.
Tucson, AZ 85733

A. W. Peller & Associates
Educational Materials
249 Goffle Road
Hawthorne, NJ 07507

Opportunities for Learning, Inc.
8950 Lurline Ave., Dep. L5869
Chatsworth, CA 91311

Merit Computer Resource Centre
3701 NW 50th
Oklahoma City, OK 73112

Reston Publishing Company
% Prentice Hall
Englewood Cliffs, NJ 07632

Gamco Industries, Inc.
P. O. Box 310
Big Spring, TX 79721

Parrot Software
190 Sandy Ridge Road
State College, PA 16801

C. C. Publications, Inc.
P. O. Box 23699
Tigard, OR 97223

Sunset Software
11750 Sunset Blvd., Suite 414
Los Angeles, CA 90049

Chas. Merrill Publishing Co.
Test Division
1300 Alum Creek Drive
Columbus, OH 43216

DLM/Teaching Resources
P. O. Box 4000
Allen, TX 75002

Hartley Courseware, Inc.
Cognitive Rehabilitation Series
123 Bridge
Dimondale, MI 48821

Cognitive Rehabilitation Series
Speech & Language Pathology
Wm. Beaumont Hospital
3601 West 13 Mile Road
Royal Oak, MI 48072

LinguiSystems, Inc.
1630 Fifth Ave., Suite 806
Moline, IL 61265

Clinical Software Resources
2850 Windemere
Birmingham, MI 48008

Computer Learning Materials Inc.
P. O. Box 1325
Ann Arbor, MI 48106

Brain-Link Software
317 Montgomery
Ann Arbor, MI 48103

Schneier Communication Unit
Cerebral Palsy Center
1603 Court Street
Syracuse, NY 13208

Southern Micro Systems
P. O. Box 2097
Burlington, NC 27216

Computer Ass't Rehab (CARE)
1121 Richwood Avenue
Cincinnati, OH 45226

Follet Library Book, Co.
4506 Northwest Highway
Crystal Lake, IL 60014

Harding & Harris
Box 1599
Orem, UT 84057

Audio Cybernetics Limited
460 California Avenue
Palo Alto, CA 94306

Learning Tools Inc.
686 Massachusetts Ave.
Cambridge, MA 02139

The Speech Bin
8 Beechtree Lane
Plainsboro, NJ 08536

Micro Video
314 N. First Street
P. O. Box 7357
Ann Arbor, MI 48107

Microcomputer Applications
RD #2, Box 229
Selinsgrove, PA 17870

Maico Hearing Instruments
7375 Bush Lake Road
Minneapolis, MN 55435

AND/OR Corporation
2801 Youngfield
Golden, CO 80401

RC Electronics
5386-D Hollister Avenue
Santa Barbara, CA 93111

Dormac, Inc.
P. O. Box 1699
Beaverton, OR 97075

College-Hill Press
4284 41st Street
San Diego, CA 92105

Appendix C: Lingquest Analysis

LINGQUEST 1

COMPUTER - ASSISTED LANGUAGE SAMPLE ANALYSIS

Dennis R. Mordecai, Ph.D.
Michael W. Palin, M.A.
and
Cheryl B. Palmer, M.S.

Client   : JOHN DOE   Birthdate : 4/4/44   C.A. : 40

Address   : 111 OAK STREET   Date of Sample : 9/9/84

           : MOBILE AL   School/Facility : POSTDOC

Clinician : JLF   Grade   : ADVANCED

LANGUAGE SAMPLE

1
```
art adj cop adj
THE BOY IS  RUNNING
THE BOY IS  RUNNING
art adj cop adj
```

2
```
pers adj     prep art adj
WE   STAYED AT   THE RANCH
WE   STAYED AT   THE RANCH
pers adj     prep art adj
```

3
```
adv cop indf pos adj
NOW IS  IT   MY  TURN
NOW IS  IT   MY  TURN
adv cop indf pos adj
```

4
```
adj  prep art  adj   prep pers
GO   TO   THE  STORE FOR  ME
ME   GO   TO   THE   STORE
pers adj  prep art   adj
```

5
```
adv cop  art  adj   prep quant adj  N+s prep inf  prep art adj prep pos   adj
NOW IS   THE  TIME  FOR  ALL   GOOD MEN TO   COME TO   THE AID OF   THEIR PARTY
MEN COME TO   PARTY
N+s V+d  prep adj                            inf
```

```
                    LEXICAL ANALYSIS
                    ----------------


        EXPANDED                CLIENT
        --------                ------

        AID             1 X -> Ø
        ALL             1 X -> Ø
        AT              1 X -> AT
        BOY             1 X -> BOY
        COME            1 X -> Ø
        FOR             1 X -> Ø
        FOR             1 X -> STORE
        GO              1 X -> ME
        GOOD            1 X -> Ø
        IS              1 X -> COME
        IS              2 X -> IS
        IT              1 X -> IT
        ME              1 X -> Ø
        MEN             1 X -> Ø
        MY              1 X -> MY
        NOW             1 X -> MEN
        NOW             1 X -> NOW
        OF              1 X -> Ø
        PARTY           1 X -> Ø
        RANCH           1 X -> RANCH
        RUNNING         1 X -> RUNNING
        STAYED          1 X -> STAYED
        STORE           1 X -> THE
        THE             1 X -> Ø
        THE             2 X -> THE
        THE             2 X -> TO
        THEIR           1 X -> Ø
        TIME            1 X -> PARTY
        TO              2 X -> Ø
        TO              1 X -> GO
        TURN            1 X -> TURN
        WE              1 X -> WE
```

```
                    LEXICAL ANALYSIS SUMMARY
                    ------------------------
```

	TOTAL SAMPLE	FIRST FIFTY
Total number of different words used :	17	-
Total number of words used :	23	-
Type / Token Ratio :	.73	-

FORM ANALYSIS

	OPPORTUNITIES	TOTAL CORRECT	PERCENT CORRECT	TOTAL ERRORS	* OMIT	* SUBST
NOUNS						
-----						
singular nouns	0	-	-	-	-	-
plural nouns						
regular	0	-	-	-	-	-
irregular	1	0	0%	1	1	0
personal pronouns	2	1	50%	1	1	0
ME	1	0	0%	1	1	0
WE	1	1	100%	0	0	0
indefinite pronouns	1	1	100%	0	0	0
IT	1	1	100%	0	0	0
demonstrative pronouns	0	-	-	-	-	-
Wh pronouns	0	-	-	-	-	-
reflexive pronouns	0	-	-	-	-	-
gerunds	0	-	-	-	-	-
VERBS						
-----						
uninflected main verbs	0	-	-	-	-	-
present tense 3rd						
person singular verbs	0	-	-	-	-	-
present participles	0	-	-	-	-	-
past tense verbs						
regular past tense	0	-	-	-	-	-
irregular past tense	0	-	-	-	-	-
past participles						
regular past	0	-	-	-	-	-
irregular past	0	-	-	-	-	-
copulas - main verb "to be"						
present tense						
am	0	-	-	-	-	-
is	3	2	66%	1	0	1
are	0	-	-	-	-	-
present tense contracted						
'm	0	-	-	-	-	-
's	0	-	-	-	-	-
're	0	-	-	-	-	-
past tense						
was	0	-	-	-	-	-
were	0	-	-	-	-	-
auxiliaries "to be"						
present tense						
am	0	-	-	-	-	-
is	0	-	-	-	-	-
are	0	-	-	-	-	-

```
present tense contracted
        'm              0     -     -     -     -     -
        's              0     -     -     -     -     -
        're             0     -     -     -     -     -
past tense
        was             0     -     -     -     -     -
        were            0     -     -     -     -     -
        been            0     -     -     -     -     -
main verbs  "to do"
        do              0     -     -     -     -     -
        does            0     -     -     -     -     -
        did             0     -     -     -     -     -
        done            0     -     -     -     -     -
auxiliaries "to do"
        do              0     -     -     -     -     -
        does            0     -     -     -     -     -
        did             0     -     -     -     -     -
main verbs  "to have"
        have            0     -     -     -     -     -
        has             0     -     -     -     -     -
        had             0     -     -     -     -     -
auxiliaries "to have"
        uncontracted
        have            0     -     -     -     -     -
        has             0     -     -     -     -     -
        had             0     -     -     -     -     -
        contracted
        've             0     -     -     -     -     -
        's              0     -     -     -     -     -
        'd              0     -     -     -     -     -
modals                  0     -     -     -     -     -
catenatives             0     -     -     -     -     -
infinitives             1     0    0%     1     1     0


MODIFIERS
---------

articles                5     2   40%     3     1     2
              THE       5     2   40%     3     1     2
quantitatives           1     0    0%     1     1     0
              ALL       1     0    0%     1     1     0
demonstrative pronouns  0     -     -     -     -     -
possessive pronouns     2     1   50%     1     1     0
              MY        1     1  100%     0     0     0
              THEIR     1     0    0%     1     1     0
possession marker       0     -     -     -     -     -
participles             0     -     -     -     -     -
adjectives             11     5   45%     6     3     3
adverbs                 2     1   50%     1     0     1
```

```
PREPOSITIONS
------------

prepositions              7      1    14%     6    4    2
           AT             1      1   100%     0    0    0
           FOR            2      0     0%     2    1    1
           OF             1      0     0%     1    1    0
           TO             3      0     0%     3    2    1
particles                 0      -     -      -    -    -


CONJUNCTIONS
------------

conjunctions              0      -     -      -    -    -


NEGATION
--------

negation lexicon          0      -     -      -    -    -
is/am/are/was/were + not
     copula               0      -     -      -    -    -
     auxiliary            0      -     -      -    -    -
is/am/are/was/were + n't
     copula               0      -     -      -    -    -
     auxiliary            0      -     -      -    -    -
modal + not               0      -     -      -    -    -
modal + n't               0      -     -      -    -    -
do/does/did + not
     main verb            0      -     -      -    -    -
     auxiliary            0      -     -      -    -    -
do/does/did + n't
     main verb            0      -     -      -    -    -
     auxiliary            0      -     -      -    -    -
have/has/had + not
     main verb            0      -     -      -    -    -
     auxiliary            0      -     -      -    -    -
have/has/had + n't
     main verb            0      -     -      -    -    -
     auxiliary            0      -     -      -    -    -


INTERJECTIONS
-------------

exclamations              0      -     -      -    -    -
greetings                 0      -     -      -    -    -


Wh Question Words
-----------------

Wh Question Words         0      -     -      -    -    -
```

```
                              * FORM ANALYSIS
                              ----------------

                              ERROR PROFILE
                              -------------

NOUNS
-----

plural nouns
     irregular
               MEN           1 X -> Ø
personal pronouns
               ME            1 X -> Ø


VERBS
-----

present tense 3rd
past tense verbs
past participles
copulas - main verb "to be"
     present tense
          is
               IS            1 X -> COME
     present tense contracted
     past tense
auxiliaries "to be"
     present tense
     present tense contracted
     past tense
main verbs  "to do"
auxiliaries "to do"
main verbs  "to have"
auxiliaries "to have"
     uncontracted
     contracted
infinitives
               COME          1 X -> Ø


MODIFIERS
---------

articles
               THE           1 X -> Ø
               THE           2 X -> TO
quantitatives
               ALL           1 X -> Ø
```

```
possessive pronouns
           THEIR          1 X -> Ø
adjectives
           AID            1 X -> Ø
           GO             1 X -> ME
           GOOD           1 X -> Ø
           PARTY          1 X -> Ø
           STORE          1 X -> THE
           TIME           1 X -> PARTY
adverbs
           NOW            1 X -> MEN


PREPOSITIONS
------------

prepositions
           FOR            1 X -> Ø
           FOR            1 X -> STORE
           OF             1 X -> Ø
           TO             2 X -> Ø
           TO             1 X -> GO


CONJUNCTIONS
------------



NEGATION
--------

is/am/are/was/were + not
is/am/are/was/were + n't
do/does/did + not
do/does/did + n't
have/has/had + not
have/has/had + n't


INTERJECTIONS
-------------



Wh Question Words
-----------------
```

```
                    FORM ANALYSIS SUMMARY
                    ---------------------
Number of different form types that computer can identify :        81


Number of different form types that did occur :                    8

Number of different form types that had an opportunity to occur :  11


Overall percent correct form usage :
            Total number correct                          14
            ------------------------------         =  --- =   38%
            Total number of opportunities                 36




                 MEAN LENGTH OF UTTERANCE (MLU)
                 -----------------------------

                                  CLIENT     EXPANDED
                                  ------     --------

TOTAL NUMBER OF UTTERANCES          5           5
TOTAL NUMBER OF WORDS              23          36
TOTAL NUMBER OF MORPHEMES          25          37

MLU BY WORDS                      4.60        7.20
MLU BY MORPHEMES                  5.00        7.40
```

STRUCTURE ANALYSIS

	OPPORTUNITIES	TOTAL CORRECT	PERCENT CORRECT	TOTAL ERRORS
Phrase Structures				
NP	2	2	100%	0
VP	0	–	–	–
MP	0	–	–	–
Basic Sentence Structures				
VP + NP	0	–	–	–
NP + VP (+NP)	0	–	–	–
NP + cop + NP/mod	0	–	–	–
NP + aux + VP	0	–	–	–
aux + VP + NP	0	–	–	–
NP (+ aux) + cat (+ VP)	0	–	–	–
NP + modal (+ aux) + VP (+ NP)	0	–	–	–
Questions				
Rising Intonation Questions	0	–	–	–
Interrogative Reversals				
aux + NP + VP ?	0	–	–	–
cop + NP + NP/mod ?	1	1	100%	0
modal + NP + VP ?	0	–	–	–
WH-Questions				
Wh + aux + NP + VP (+ NP) ?	0	–	–	–
Wh + cop + NP/mod ?	0	–	–	–
Wh + modal + NP + VP (+ NP) ?	0	–	–	–
Wh + VP (+ NP) ?	0	–	–	–
Wh + aux + VP (+ NP) ?	0	–	–	–
Wh (+ NP) ?	0	–	–	–
Complex Sentences				
INFINITIVE	0	–	–	–
DOUBLE INFINITIVE	0	–	–	–

		TOTAL	PERCENT	TOTAL
	OPPORTUNITIES	CORRECT	CORRECT	ERRORS

COORDINATION	0	-	-	-
CONJUNCTION DELETION				
(object)	0	-	-	-
(predicate)	0	-	-	-
(subject)	0	-	-	-
ADVERBIAL CLAUSE	0	-	-	-
RELATIVE CLAUSE				
(subj. related)	0	-	-	-
(obj. related)	0	-	-	-
(pronoun deletion)	0	-	-	-
INFINITIVE CLAUSE WITH DIFFERENT SUBJECT	1	0	0%	1
Wh-INFINITIVE CLAUSE	0	-	-	-

UNIDENTIFIABLE STRUCTURES
1

CHECK THE UNIDENTIFIABLE STRUCTURES TO SEE IF
ANY ARE OF THE FOLLOWING TYPES

		TOTAL	PERCENT	TOTAL
	OPPORTUNITIES	CORRECT	CORRECT	ERRORS

EMBEDDING WITH COORDINATION

DOUBLE EMBEDDING

COMPLEX QUESTION

COMPLEX STRUCTURE COMBINATIONS

220

Appendix C

STRUCTURE ANALYSIS SUMMARY

Number of different structure types computer can identify :   32

Number of different identifiable structure types that did occur :   3

Number of different identifiable structure types
that had an opportunity to occur :   3

Number of uninflected single word utterances :   0

Overall percent correct identifiable structure usage :
            Total number correct   3
            -------------------------------   -- = 75%
            Total number of opportunities   4

VERB TENSE ANALYSIS

	OPPORTUNITIES	TOTAL CORRECT	PERCENT CORRECT	TOTAL ERRORS
Simple Present Tense	3	2	66%	1
Simple Past Tense	0	–	–	–
Simple Future Tense	0	–	–	–
Present Perfect Tense	0	–	–	–
Past Perfect Tense	0	–	–	–
Future Perfect Tense	0	–	–	–
Present Progressive Tense	0	–	–	–
Past Progressive Tense	0	–	–	–
Future Progressive Tense	0	–	–	–
Present Perfect Progressive Tense	0	–	–	–
Past Perfect Progressive Tense	0	–	–	–
Future Perfect Progressive Tense	0	–	–	–

VERB TENSE ANALYSIS SUMMARY

Number of different tenses computer can identify :   12

Number of different identifiable tenses that did occur :   1

Number of different identifiable tenses
that had an opportunity to occur :   1

Overall percent correct identifiable tense usage :

       Total number correct

$$\frac{\text{Total number correct}}{\text{Total number of opportunities}} = \frac{2}{3} = 66\%$$

Appendix D: List of Suggested Computer Periodicals

SUGGESTED PERIODICALS

A+
P. O. Box 2965
Boulder, CO 80321

Byte
P. O. Box 590
Martinsville, NJ 08836

Commodore/Power Play
Commodore Business Machines
Box 651
Holmes, PA 19043

Compute
Box 5406
Greensboro, NC 27403

Computer Shopper
Patch Publishing Company
407 S. Washington Ave.
Titusville, FL 32781

Creative Computing
P. O. Box 5214
Boulder, CO 80321

Family Computing
Box 2511
Boulder, CO 80302

Home Computer Magazine
Emerald Village Publishing
Box 70288
Eugene, OR 97401

InCider
P. O. Box 911
Farmingdale, NY 11737

Interface Age
16704 Marquardt Avenue
Cerritos, CA 90701

Mac World
Box 20300
Bergenfield, NJ 07621

Nibble Magazine
45 Winthrop Street
Concord, MA 01742

PC: The Independent Guide
      to Personal Computers
Box 2455
Boulder, CO 80322

PC World
P. O. Box 6700
Bergenfield, NJ 07621

Personal Computing
Box 2942
Boulder, CO 80322

Popular Computing
P. O. Box 328
Hancock, NH 03449

The Rainbow
9529 U. S. Highway 42
Box 385
Prospect, KY 40059

Glossary

Algorithm: A step-by-step formula for resolving a problem.

ASCII: Acronym for American Standard Code for Information Interchange. First used with teletype transmission, it is the standard code for inputting characters from the keyboard.

Baud: A unit of signaling speed. Equates to bits per second. 300 and 1200 baud are common signaling speeds for modem information transmission.

BASIC: Acronym for Beginner's All-Purpose Symbolic Instruction Code. BASIC was developed at Dartmouth College in 1963 and is the most popular language for microcomputer programming.

Binary: Base two system in numbers. Consists of the characters *0* and *1*. All internal computations in the computer are done in binary math.

Bit: Smallest unit of coding for the computer. The code is binary, so the bit is represented by a *0* or *1*. In reality, a bit is a stored electrical state.

Boot: To start. Cold boot refers to turning the computer on. Warm boot refers to restarting the initial system program once a computer is on.

Buffer: Storage area for information. Buffers hold information being input until the device to which it is being input can process it. Buffers allow information to be "dumped" (entered) from the computer to a device, such as a printer. By doing this, the computer does not have to wait for the printer and is free for other tasks.

Bug: Error either in hardware or software.

Byte: Basic unit of information for computer processing. Consists of a set number of bits, depending on the computer, that are processed simultaneously. Eight-bit and 16-bit computers are most common.

Character: Symbol which is input to the computer. Normally it is input as an ASCII code.

Central processing unit: A single IC (integrated circuit) chip which performs operations and directs the flow of information and instructions within the computer. In the microcomputer the chip is called the *microprocessor.*

Compiler: Type of language that takes instructions written in symbolic code and translates them into machine language. The advantage of compiled languages is that they execute quickly.

CRT: Abbreviation for cathode ray tube, which is the principal component of the monitor.

File: Information that is formatted in such a way that it can be stored or retrieved by the computer from a storage device.

Graphic: Display of dots in any form, either on a monitor or a printer.

Hardware: Any tangible part of a computer system, as opposed to software, which is a set of instructions that control the operation of a computer.

Hexadecimal: Base 16 system. Often used to specify computer values. Consists of characters 0, 1, 2, 3, 4, 5, 6, 7, 8, 9, A, B, C, D, E, and F.

Input: (Noun) Device which transmits information to the computer. (Verb) Process of transmitting information to the computer.

Instruction: Statement executed by the computer.

Integrated circuit: Thin wafer (chip) of a silicon which contains an electronic circuit. An unlimited number of circuits, which can only be seen with magnification, can be put on a single chip.

Interface: A connection between two hardware components so that they can communicate. Communication may be serial (bit by bit) or parallel (byte by byte).

Kilobyte: Abbreviated K, it means 1024 bytes. Memory and storage capacity is usually expressed in kilobytes, e.g., 64K computer, 360K disk drive.

Machine language: Code in which the computer actually stores information and carries out instructions. Normally the code is binary.

Memory: Amount of information that can be stored in a device. Dynamic memory refers to the amount of information that can be stored at one time in the computer, but is lost when the computer is turned off. Passive memory refers to the amount of information that can be stored for retrieval, through devices such as cassettes, floppy disks, and hard disks.

Microcomputer: Computer which can sit on a desk top and operates through a single chip called a *microprocessor.*

Microprocessor: Integrated circuit chip that controls the operation of a microcomputer. It sequences and executes instructions stored in memory, accepts information from inputs, and generates code to output devices as programmed.

Modem: A hardware device that allows information to be exchanged between two computers using the telephone. The name is derived from its function, which is modulation and demodulation of the signal.

Operating system: Also called disk operating system (DOS). System of instructions for controlling disk operations. The most common present systems are MS DOS (IBM PC), Apple DOS 3.3 (Apple II/IIe/IIc), and C/PM (generic to computers with Z80 (or compatible) microprocessors).

Parallel transmission: Information transmitted in bytes, i.e., several bits simultaneously.

Program: Set of instructions which controls the operation of a computer.

PROM: Programmable read-only memory. Chips with ROM which can be reprogrammed with special equipment.

ROM: Read-only memory. IC chips with programs or information permanently stored on them. These cannot be changed by the operator.

Real-time clock: Clock interfaced with computer which keeps time to the fraction of a second. It is powered by a battery when the computer is not on to maintain time from operation to operation.

Real-time process: Operation which occurs as the event being processed happens. Real-time analysis refers to analysis of data at the time at which data is received (as opposed to data that is stored and later retrieved for analysis).

RS232C: An industry standard for serial transmission of data.

Serial transmission: Transmission of data bit by bit (as opposed to parallel transmission).

Software: Set of instructions which controls the operation of a computer.

Source code: A printed set of instructions given the computer. The source code can be in a language (e. g., BASIC, FORTRAN, PASCAL, C language), or it can be coded in terms of assembly language.

Subroutine: A small, self-contained program that can be called to be used in the main program. Subroutines are usually instruction sequences that are carried out several times during the administration of a program. By calling them up as a subroutine, the set of instructions does not have to be rewritten in the main program each time.

Syntax: The rules governing the use of symbols of a language.

Text: Standard computer characters, such as letters, numbers, and special characters as !a#$%&*()-+. As opposed to graphics.

Index